Cheryl Waites, EdD, MSW
Editor

Social Work Practice with African-American Families
An Intergenerational Perspective

Pre-publication
REVIEWS,
COMMENTARIES,
EVALUATIONS . . .

"**O**ffers a critical perspective to the social work profession for working with African-American Families. . . . The contributors to this volume, utilizing the intergenerational perspective, present refreshing, innovative, and practical methods of working with African-American families to help them help themselves. . . . Although this volume focuses particularly on African-American families, an intergenerational perspective will lend itself to families of other races and ethnicities."

Bernita C. Berry, PhD, MSW
Associate Professor and Chair,
Department of Social Work,
Savannah State University

"**T**imely and important . . . filled with insights, program examples, and practice approaches connecting the past to the present . . . provides an intergenerational, strengths-based perspective on working with African-American families. From the richness of the voices resonating from its pages a comprehensive framework for culturally competent, contextualized, social justice-based practice emerges. Each chapter identifies how families draw on the assets that are passed down to people through time and shows us how practitioners can extract power, resilience, and capital from past and current intergenerational relationships and traditions to tackle the unique twenty-first century challenges facing African-American families and communities. . . . A must-read; an invaluable resource for all social workers and other helping professionals."

Dorothy Van Soest, PhD, MSW
Professor, University of Washington, Seattle

Social Work Practice with African-American Families
An Intergenerational Perspective

SOCIAL WORK PRACTICE IN ACTION
Edited by
Marvin D. Feit, The University of Akron in Ohio, USA.

Also available in the series:

Social Work Practice with African-American Families

An Intergenerational Perspective

Cheryl Waites, EdD, MSW
Editor

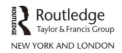 Routledge
Taylor & Francis Group

NEW YORK AND LONDON

First published 2008
by Routledge
270 Madison Ave, New York, NY 10016

Simultaneously published in the UK
by Routledge
2 Park Square, Milton Park, Abingdon, Oxon OX14 4RN

Routledge is an imprint of the Taylor & Francis Group, an informa business

Printed and bound in the United States of America on acid-free paper
by Edwards Brothers, Inc.

Library of Congress Cataloging-in-Publication Data
Social work practice with African American families : an
intergenerational perspective / [edited
by] Cheryl Waites.
p. cm.
Includes bibliographical references.
ISBN: 978-0-7890-3391-8 (hard : alk. paper)
ISBN: 978-0-7890-3392-5 (soft : alk. paper)
1. Social work with African Americans. I. Waites, Cheryl.
HV3181.S613 2007
362.84'96073—dc22
2007039821

ISBN 10: 0-7890-3391-7 (hbk)
ISBN 10: 0-7890-3392-5 (pbk)

ISBN 13: 978-0-7890-3391-8 (hbk)
ISBN 13: 978-0-7890-3392-5 (pbk)

CONTENTS

ABOUT THE EDITOR

Cheryl Waites, EdD, MSW, is an associate professor and associate dean of the School of Social Work, at Wayne State University. She received her BA in sociology from Hunter College (CUNY), her MSW from Fordham University, and her EdD in counselor education from North Carolina State University. Dr. Waites is a Hartford Faculty Scholar. Her areas of research include healthy aging, health disparities, intergenerational relationships, and culturally appropriate and responsive practice. She has also studied promising practices for enhancing gerontological social work education and training. Dr. Waites received a grant from the Institute of Geriatric Social Work at Boston University and conducted a capacity-building project to provide training opportunities for practitioners interested in developing competencies in working with older adults and their families. She was also a recipient of a Geriatric Enrichment in Social Work Education grant, sponsored by the John A. Hartford Foundation and the Council on Social Work Education. She instituted and evaluated an educational change process designed to infuse aging content across the social work curricula. Dr. Waites has received several other grants in the areas of family-centered practice, cultural competency, and social work education. Dr. Waites has numerous publications in refereed journals, and has written several book chapters, teaching/training books, and technical reports. Dr. Waites has also presented her research at numerous international, national, and regional conferences.

CONTRIBUTORS

Kilolo Brodie, MSW, is currently the Title IV-E Project Coordinator at California State University East Bay in the Social Work Department. Ms. Brodie has worked as a county child welfare worker in California, and for community collaboratives in Washington, DC, as a family group conference coordinator and facilitator. She has also taught foundation, and advanced master's and bachelor's level social work courses. Ms. Brodie is a PhD candidate at Howard University School of Social Work.

Iris B. Carlton-LaNey, PhD, is a professor in the School of Social Work at the University of North Carolina at Chapel Hill. She received her BSW from North Carolina A&T State University, her MA from the University of Chicago, and her PhD from the University of Maryland at Baltimore. Her research interests include aging in rural communities and African-American social welfare history. She has served as guest editor for special issues of the *Journal of Sociology and Social Welfare* and the *Journal of Community Practice* (along with Dr. N. Y. Burwell), and has authored a monograph titled *Elderly Black Farm Women As Keepers of the Community and Culture.* She has served on the editorial boards of several journals and has published articles in *Affilia, Arete, Generations,* the *Journal of Community Practice,* the *Journal of Sociology & Social Welfare, Social Service Review,* and *Social Work.* Dr. Carlton-LaNey has co-edited two books, *African American Community Practice Models Historical and Contemporary Responses* (with Dr. N. Y. Burwell), and *Preserving and Strengthening Small Towns and Rural Communities* (with Drs. R. L. Edwards and P. N. Reid). In 2001 the National Association of Social Workers Press published *African American Leadership: An Empowerment Tradition in Social Welfare History.* Dr. Carlton-LaNey has lectured on African-American social welfare history and African Americans aging in the rural south at several schools of social work across the country. She has recently (2005) published a book titled *African Americans Aging in the Rural South: Stories of Faith, Family and Community.*

Deidre Helen Crumbley, PhD, is Associate Professor of Africana Studies in the Interdisciplinary Studies Division of North Carolina State University. Trained as a sociocultural anthropologist, her research focuses on gender, power, and religious change in Africa and its North American diaspora. Her forthcoming book, *Sprit, Structure and Flesh: Gender and Power in African Instituted Churches (AICs),* investigates the interplay of gender, power, doctrine, and ritual in the rise and development of AICs. Her current book project is a historically embedded ethnography of a female founded inner-city storefront church, paying special attention to the place of gender, race, and migration in religious community formation and sustainability.

Molly Everett Davis, EdD, is Associate Professor, and Director of the BSW Field Education in the Department of Social Work at George Mason University. She received a BA in psychology from Louisiana State University, her MSW from Tulane University, and her EdD in Higher Education Administration from Florida State University. Dr. Davis' areas of research include mental health practice and policy, intergenerational theory and practice, gerontology, cultural competence models, and social work education. She is the recipient of a number of grants on community development with at risk families. Dr. Davis has presented her work in research and theoretical models to national and international conferences. She is the author of a number of book chapters, articles, manuals, and research reports.

Charnetta Gadling-Cole, MSW, is the founder and executive director of Just For Me, Inc. and is president of J&J Consultants, LLC. Ms. Gadling-Cole earned her BA in psychology from Johnson C. Smith University, MSW from the University of South Carolina (Columbia) and is presently a PhD candidate at Howard University School of Social Work specializing in gerontology and public policy. She has served as a fellow at the National Institute of Health, conducted international qualitative research in Nairobi, Kenya, for HIV/ AIDS Caregivers. She has successfully developed programs and policies and written grants for various nonprofit organizations. She is currently conducting needs assessment for people living with HIV and AIDS and their caregivers in Haiti and South Africa. She has also published on utilizing family group conferences for work with older adults and their caregivers.

Monica Terrell Leach, holds a BS from Louisiana State University, an MEd and EdD in higher education administration from North Carolina State University (NCSU). Currently, she is Assistant Professor in the Department of Social Work and Assistant Dean for Academic Affairs in the College of Humanities and Social Sciences at NCSU. Her research interests include social work and education; the academic achievement gap as it relates to college-age students; and the relationship between schools and families in promoting academic success for poor and minority children. She is very active in the community, serving on several boards and foundations.

Bernice W. Liddie-Hamilton, PhD, is Associate Adjunct Professor of the Whitney M. Young Jr. School of Medicine, Clark Atlanta University and Morehouse School of Medicine in Atlanta, Georgia. She previously chaired special work programs at Marymount College Tarrytown, Benedict College, and the Whitney M. Young Jr. School of Social Work. She holds a BA in psychology, nursing, and social work from Pace University, Marymount College Tarrytown, Columbia University and Fordham University. Dr. Liddie-Hamilton is a recipient of a Fulbright-Hayes scholarship to study and work in the Dominican Republic. Her research interests and scholarship include policy issues related to race and ethnic relations, welfare reform, health and ethics, publications in several journal articles, chapters, and presentations at numerous national conferences.

Annie McCullough-Chavis, EdD, is Associate Professor of Social Work and Director of Field Education in the Master of Social Work Program at Fayetteville State University. She received her BA in sociology and social studies with honors from Fayetteville State University and the MSW from the School of Social Work at the University of North Carolina at Chapel Hill. She obtained the EdD in educational leadership from Fayetteville State University. Dr. Chavis has nineteen years of teaching experience on the university level as an undergraduate and graduate faculty. Her research interests include family genograms and assessment, intervention with African-American families, student mentoring, and cultural competence. She has published journal articles on the genograms and has lectured and presented on the genograms and family assessment at several universities, and local, state, regional, and national conferences.

Elijah Mickel, DSW, CRT, LICSW, is Professor and Acting Chair of the Social Work Department, Assistant Dean of the College of Health and Public Policy at Delaware State University. He earned a DSW and an MSW from Howard University, and a Masters of Adult Education, Supervision and Administration from the University of the District of Columbia. His current research areas include mental health, family welfare, and higher education leadership. He has developed a beginning body of literature in the area of African-centered reality therapy and choice theory. Dr. Mickel has written a book titled *African Centered Reality Therapy.* In addition, he has also developed a body of literature dealing with the contributions of African Americans to the development of self-help, social and economic justice, and liberation.

Dorothy S. Ruiz, PhD, is Associate Professor of African Studies and Sociology at the University of North Carolina at Charlotte. Dr. Ruiz received her PhD from Michigan State University in sociology. Her research focuses on caregiving among African-American grandmothers. She examines health and social indicators of depression, stress, and life satisfaction among caregiving grandmothers. In addition, she has explored the impact of mental health and mental disorder in African-American populations. Among her major contributions are two books: *The Handbook of Mental Health and Mental Disorders Among Black Americans* (Greenwood, 1991), and *Amazing Grace: African American Grandmothers As Caregivers and Conveyers of Traditional Values* (Praeger, 2004).

Andrea Stewart, DSW, is Professor and director of the Social Work Program at the University of Arkansas at Pine Bluff. She received her BA in sociology from the University of Arkansas at Little Rock, her MSW from the University of Arkansas at Little Rock, and her DSW from Howard University. A consultant and volunteer to a variety of private and public agencies, Dr. Stewart has also served on a number of boards, task forces, and committees at both the national and local levels. Her most recent publication includes a book chapter titled "Truth and Consequences: My Personal Story As a Woman of Color" in *Women of Color As Social Work Educators: Strengths and Survival.* Dr. Stewart's research interests include teenage pregnancy issues, single parenting, aging, youth programming, and spirituality. She has received more than $3.5 million in grants and contracts.

Jocelyn DeVance Taliaferro, PhD, is Assistant Professor in the North Carolina State University Department of Social Work. Dr. Taliaferro has a PhD in urban affairs and public policy from the University of Delaware. Her research interests are nonprofit organizations, community development, urban poverty, and program/policy evaluation. She currently teaches community practice and research design and methodology courses for the Department of Social Work. Dr. Taliaferro has published in such journals as *Journal of Human Behavior in the Social Environment* and *Journal of Family Social Work.* In addition, Dr. Taliaferro has more than a decade of professional experience in the nonprofit sector and the field of social work, which includes the position of executive director of the Black Mental Health Alliance for Education and Consultation, Inc., and business manager of People Encouraging People, Inc. (a nonprofit, vocational rehabilitation organization). Dr. Taliaferro has also served as the chairperson for the Baltimore City Mayor's Mental Health Advisory Committee.

Makeba Thomas, PhD, is Assistant Professor at Bowie State University. She has earned a PhD from Clark-Atlanta University, and an MSW from Howard University. Her current research area is centered on African-American women and addiction. Dr. Thomas has presented her research at several conferences including the NIH Conference on Understanding and Reducing Health Disparities, the Conference for the Dissemination of Research on Addictions, Infectious Disease, and Public Health at the Johns Hopkins School of Public Health, and most recently at the 2007 Minority Women's Health Summit in Washington, DC.

Laurie B. Welch, LMSW, holds a BS in psychology from the University of Illinois, Urbana-Champaign and an MSW from the University of Houston Graduate College of Social Work. Currently, she works in Houston, Texas, as a children's therapist at DePelchin Children's Center. She is employed within the Residential Treatment Program at DePelchin, where she specializes in experiential and recreational therapies. Her clinical and research interests include the developmental effects of childhood trauma, the differential impact of peer victimization in males versus females, and the use of experiential and recreational therapies with child and adolescent trauma victims.

Sheara A. Williams, MSW, PhD, ACSW, is Assistant Professor at the University of Houston Graduate College of Social Work, where she teaches practice and school social work courses. Her research interests and activities focus on children's behavioral and emotional health in school settings; the psychosocial factors that impact the academic achievement of minority children, particularly African-American and Hispanic/Latino youths; and family-school interventions that promote school readiness and school success for poor and minority children. In addition, Dr. Williams facilitates cultural awareness and sensitivity workshops and has a culmination of eight years of practice experience with substance-using juvenile offenders, inner-city youths, medical/mental health social work, and educational attainment.

Acknowledgments

I wish to thank my contributors for the wonderful work they put into preparing their chapters for this volume.

PART I:
THE INTERGENERATIONAL
PERSPECTIVE

This book will present an intergenerational approach for working with families and prepare social work students for competent practice with African-American families. Practice principles and the intergenerational perspective will provide a framework for exploring (1) the strength and resource richness of intergenerational relationships; (2) the roles and contributions of African-American elders, middle-aged adults, and children to family life; (3) the issues and challenges facing African-American multigenerational families and the extended family network; and (4) the impact of community intergenerational transactions.

Chapter 1

African-American Families Across Generations

Cheryl Waites

Family must look out for family.

African Proverb

As you look across time and generations, it is important to acknowledge the significance of multigenerational family networks and intergenerational relationships that are central to the African-American experience. History tells us that extended family networks have always been prevalent in the African diasporas. Multigenerational families (four or five generations) providing support and care for family members and fictive kin (nonblood relatives) across the life course has been well documented (Billingsley, 1992, 1999; Freeman & Logan, 2004; Hill, 1972, 1999; Ladner, 1998; Logan, 2001; McAdoo, 1997; McCubbin, 1998; Staples, 1999; Taylor, Jackson, & Chatters, 1997). Equally established are the reports of family and community perseverance in the face of disparity and oppressions spanning 400 years of slavery, years of "Jim Crow," decades of segregation, marginalization, and continued intentional and unintentional racism (Christian, 1995). In spite of these barriers, there is a legacy of people of African descent with strong family connections, resilience, spirituality, and hope (Bagley & Carroll, 1998; Denby, 1996).

A deficit model—problem-focused approach—is sometimes used to understand African-American families who have carried on in often

Social Work Practice with African-American Families

hostile environments. This approach neither considers the resilience and achievements of African Americans across time and generations, nor does it attempt to understand and build on these successes and strengths. It is paramount that social workers, and other professionals, appreciate family and community strengths and the pathways that lead to triumph over adversity. This involves understanding the legacies and traditions of the African-American families and communities as well as the structural constraints, the historical realities, and the overall cultural context across time and generations (Barnes, 2001).

This chapter introduces an intergenerational, strengths-oriented perspective. A strengths perspective emphasizes the capacities and competencies of clients (Saleebey, 1992) while acknowledging the social context. An intergenerational perspective recognizes strengths, challenges, and transactions across time and generations. However, it fundamentally serves as a lens that provides multidimensional life course information, insight, history, and traditions. Cross-generational strengths—generational legacies that have been transmitted across generations—intergenerational transmissions, and current cultural context all are significant to this perspective. An intergenerational approach provides a framework for discussing the past, the current context, and promising practices that may be helpful for work with African-American families from older adult to youth. To fully understand and utilize an intergenerational perspective it is important to understand and connect with the past and the social-historical understanding that lays the foundation for this approach.

RICH TRADITIONS:
PAST AND CURRENT CONTEXTS

Understanding African-American families requires an appreciation of the realities that have shaped their experience across time, generations, and context. Enduring oppression and pervasive cutoffs from the African cultural heritage and customs, African-American families have demonstrated powerful endurance. Family practices, beliefs, and customs as well as social-political action have historically been part of African-American life. Traditions linked to spirituality, special care for children and elders, kinship ties, oral storytelling, collectivism, and unity are connected with the past and present (Barnes, 2001).

Hill (1972, 1999) has eloquently written about five assets of African-American families: strong achievement orientation, strong work orientation, flexible family roles, strong kinship bonds, and strong religious orientation. Hill and others point to strengths that are linked to history, culture, values, and adaptations and suggest that building on these strengths is a good strategy for working with African-American families (Freeman & Logan, 2004; Logan, 2001; McAdoo, 1997; McCubbin, 1998; Staples, 1999). In order to understand the multigenerational connections and intergenerational relationships one must understand these family and community strengths and traditions across time and place.

Kin Keeping

Kin keeping is a tradition in the African-American community where families are often multigenerational networks, and blood relatives and fictive kin interact across the life span to provide assistance and care. The orientation where family takes precedence over the individual is well documented (Billingsley, 1992; Hill, 1999; Hines & Boyd-Franklin, 1996). Boyd-Franklin (1989, 2003) concludes that reciprocity, the process of helping each other and exchanging and sharing support as well as goods and services, is a central part of the lives of African Americans. This principle compels one to give back to their family and community in return for what had been given to them (Sudarkasa, 1997). African Americans place a high premium on mutual assistance and interdependence; it remains an important value (Billingsley, 1999; Hill, 1999). This is evident in the prevalence of the extended family network, where adult members experience a collective social, financial, and ethical responsibility to care for family members.

African-American grandparents caring for their grandchildren and other relatives are viewed as a cultural strength (McAdoo, 2002; Scannapieco & Jackson, 1996). Well documented are examples of grandmothers, and in some cases grandfathers, who care for grandchildren whose parents are experiencing a host of social problems that hinder parenting (Cox, 2002). Grandparents, particularly grandmothers, play a central role in African-American extended families (Billingsley, 1992, 1999). They serve as guardians and caretakers for children, grandchildren, parents, extended family members, and fictive kin. Grandparents represent wisdom and strength and are the key keepers of family values such as respect, religion, love, support, and community. Grandparents, especially grandmothers, are serving more frequently as surrogate parents owing to an increase in single and adolescent parenting, divorce, crime, HIV/AIDS, and drug usage (Barnes, 2001; Ruiz & Carlton-LaNey, 1999) and this has created stress on this invaluable resource. Often these middle-aged adults are responsible for several generations, including their children, nieces and nephews, as well as parents and other elder family members (Ruiz & Carlton-LaNey, 1999). Grandparents and other kin keepers assume roles of caretaking and must prepare grandchildren to avoid pitfalls of gang activity, illegal gang involvement, premature sexual activity, negative interactions with law enforcement officers, and problems with the school system.

Gibson (2005), in discussing the parenting strategies of African-American grandparents, found that they use seven strengths:

1. maintain effective communication;
2. take a strong role in the education of their grandchildren;
3. provide socioeconomic support;
4. involve extended family;
5. involve grandchildren in selective community activities;
6. acknowledge and work with the vulnerabilities of grandchildren; and
7. deal with the absence of the biological parents.

She concludes that the Afrocentric perspective views intergenerational parenting as a potential resource and should be considered in assessing kinship care and other community resources. Older adults (age sixty and above) also play a significant role in family life by supporting younger family members, mentoring, volunteering in the community, church leadership, and participation in fraternal and civic organizations. Gibson (2005) encourages professionals to build upon the strengths of intergenerational parenting and older adults who will come forward to assume a variety of caregiving roles.

As adult children become middle aged, they may become more involved in caring for parents, grandparents, and aging relatives. The health and economic disparities of many African-American elders put them at risk for hypertension, diabetes, chronic illnesses and disability, and low wealth. A lifetime of hard work followed by poor health as they age often makes the supportive care of extended family important. Black elders are less likely to be placed in nursing homes or long-term care facilities (Hooyman & Kiyak, 2005; Taylor, Chatters, & Celious, 2003). However, some identify that this may be changing and is discussed later in this book. A variety of arrangements for the support and care of older adults can be found in the African-American community. This might include relative care of childless elders, coresidence of adult children and parents, family care to maintain elders in their home, and placement in a long-term care facility.

Oral Traditions and Intergenerational Transmissions

The African-American rich oral history has transmitted the wisdom of grandmothers and grandfathers from generation to generation and has historically helped families adapt to the realities of daily life (Carlton-LaNey, 2003, 2005; Stack, 1996, 1997). Stories and lessons learned enable all of us to step into the world and gain a glimpse of life, with all of its reality. Knowing about relationships across generations, the way families function, their church service, and the black church community cohesiveness and community traditions facilitate a deeper understanding of the cultural context and the overall environment across time and place. Oral history helps us gain insight, perspective, and cultural information. Many stories tell one of times past and link struggle, resilience, and lessons learned. They are fables often grounded in spirituality, faith, instruction, and healing (lessons for the mind, body, and soul).

Contemporary accounts of African-American families are as poignant as those from generations past. The examples of resilience and strength are just as meaningful. Families face heartbreaking difficulty, often fueled by the widespread use of drugs and the rampant spread of HIV/AIDS. Crack, in the 1980s and 1990s, put a strain on the kin support networks as many became addicted and the drug dominated their lives (Dunlap, Golub, Johnson, & Wesley, 2002; Dunlap, Golub, & Johnson, 2006). Grandparents raising grandchildren, intergenerational connections/solidarity, caregiving needs of older adults, and the rising economic and health disparities have all been exacerbated by the changing environments in the African-American diaspora and larger society as a whole.

Religion, Spirituality, and the Black Church

Religion and spiritual beliefs are the foundation of inner strength and continue to be important in the lives of African-American families (Barnes, 2001). These provide a protective factor for families when faced with the often harsh realities of daily life. The black church has played a historical role in the African-American community and has guided the community through two major reformations: the abolition of slavery and the abolition of legal racial apartheid (Jim Crow and the Civil Rights Movement) (Billingsley & Morrison-Rodriguez, 1998). Churches provide a variety of support and leadership and many families turn to the church during difficult times.

Older adults play an important role in black churches. They, especially women, are preservers of church tradition. They support the church by tidying it up, service attendance, and loyalty. They are more likely to internalize the teachings and engage in activities beyond Sunday services (Taylor & Chatters, 1989). To encourage prayers and visitations to housebound or frail members, many black churches publish weekly lists of those who are shut in because of illness or old-age related impairments. Studies have found that one out of five members received financial assistance, goods and services, or total support from the church (Lincoln & Mamiya, 1990; Taylor & Chatters, 1989). Sometimes collection plates are passed around to aid members in times of need. Some churches provide transportation services to churches, grocery shopping, and other activities. Some churches have also used U.S. Department of Housing and Urban Development Grants or congregational funds or other combinations to purchase land and provide safe and affordable housing to its disabled and elder members.

The church is a prominent institution in the black community. Yet, there have been some criticism. Many have called for the black church to take action to protect and promote health among its families through concerted action on multiple levels; to "mount a spiritual and political campaign to save African-American families, thereby ensuring their prosperity" (Billingsley & Morrison-Rodriguez, 1998). Others point to how slow the church was to respond to the HIV/AIDS. Some churches are now playing a role in intervention and prevention of this disease by acknowledging the urgency for action after realizing the life-threatening effects caused.

The Balm In Gilead, Inc., is a not-for-profit, nongovernmental organization whose mission is to "improve the health status of people of the African diaspora by building the capacity of faith communities to address life-threatening diseases, especially HIV/AIDS" (The Balm In Gilead, 2007, http://www.balmingilead.org/about/mission.asp). This group has been instrumental in advancing HIV/AIDS ministries models in the African-American churches. Two models that have been promoted since 1993 and 1989, respectively, are the Black Church National Day of Prayer for the Healing of AIDS and the Annual Harlem Week of Prayer for the Healing of AIDS. These models emphasize prevention of HIV transmission—through prayer, education, and mobilization of clergy and congregations, and are examples of intergenerational faith-based programming.

There have been some questions concerning whether the church, or the existing family social support networks, can adapt in time to meet the needs of the vast number of African-American youths who are in trouble and/or at risk. In their search for meaning and survival, significant numbers of youths are involved in risky behaviors, and some are also turning to gangs and illegal activities. This generation needs special support to ensure their survival and to maximize their potential to thrive.

A pilot study (Coyne-Beasley & Schoenbach, 2000) surveyed a convenience sample of clergy leaders from African-American churches about their young adolescent members. The survey asked about priority health topics, prevalence of sexual and drug-risk behaviors, and the clergy's desire for health education programs. The churches were located in a county (the population in 1990 was approximately 200,000, 40 percent African Americans) in the southeastern United States. The respondents' highest priority issues were drugs, violence, HIV/AIDS, pregnancy, and alcohol. Many (76 percent) had discussed one or more of these issues in church. All respondents wanted additional health seminars for their adolescents, though some clergy (30 percent) excluded some sexual topics (i.e., anal sex, bisexuality, homosexuality, masturbation, oral sex). Only 6 percent would make condoms available in their churches, but all would allow contraceptive education. Many African-American churches are open to including sex education among their health education programs for young adolescents.

For some youths, gangs have replaced their loyalty to their parents, brothers, sisters, and grandparents. Imprisonment is an inevitable consequence when engaged in illicit street life. However, few African-American congregations are involved in prison ministries, and over half of prison inmates in many prisons have not received visits from their families or friends (Lincoln & Mamiya, 1990). A generation of adolescents and young adults, particularly males, are in need of intergenerational helping systems and the church seems to be a traditional starting point.

African-American churches are among the institutions that can combat gaps in education, income, and health between blacks and whites. Franklin (2007, p. 7), states, "Black churches face a mission crisis as they struggle to serve their upwardly mobile and/or established middle class paying customers alongside the poorest of the poor." He goes on to recommend that black churches work together on specific problems facing black communities in order to deal with the "unfinished business" of helping people in need. Franklin recommends that houses of worship from different denominations collaborate to ameliorate one area of life for black Americans. He suggests, for example, that Baptist denominations specifically deal with prisoner reentry as Methodists revitalize educational efforts and Pentecostals work on youth programs. He goes on to state that "churches can and should work with other houses of worship, with local police departments and secular youth organizations to protect and redirect at-risk youth."

Walls and Zarit's (1991) study of churches indicate that the family network is perceived as more supportive than the church network, but that church support contributes to feelings of well-being. Findings from studies suggest that serving older adults is not a top priority for most congregations. Most senior programs are small and often informal (Cnaan, Boddie, & Kang, 2005). This may be an untapped resource for intergenerational helping. The black church is an underutilized resource that, if understood by professionals, can be used to enhance services to the elderly (Morrison, 1991)

Health and Well-Being: Mind, Body, and Soul

Health across generations is of concern. African Americans disproportionately suffer the ill effects of chronic illness such as hypertension, diabetes, and shorter life expectancy (Min, 2005). Historically, health and well-being in the African-American diaspora can be linked to the Atlantic slave trade during the nineteenth century and the devastating health effects it had on Africans and African Americans (Byrd & Clayton, 2000). Slave health deficits were perpetuated by the Jim Crow era and continue even today in terms of access to quality care and lack of trust of the health care system (Byrd & Clayton, 2000).

CULTURE AND CONTEXT

The Civil Rights Movement, a powerful vehicle for advocacy and social change, was followed by the "hip-hop" generation. This generational influence has grown to encompass a whole culture, lifestyle, and ideology, a point of view. Hip-hop has more influence today with young people than the Civil Rights Movement. Sometimes this contributes to generational rifts and misunderstanding. Strategies to prevent intergenerational "culture wars" (Boyd, 2004) and to build intergenerational connections need to be explored. Preserving intergenerational transmission, relationships, and collaborations is important to continued progress for African-American families and communities.

In regard to generational transmissions of values and context, Schiele (2005) identifies and examines how cultural oppression has produced three risk factors—(1) cultural estrangement, (2) attenuation of black collectivism, and (3) spiritual alienation—that diminish African-Americans' ability to advance and prosper in the United States. He indicates that these factors place African Americans at high risk of experiencing continued obstacles toward group affirmation and empowerment. Being unaware and unappreciative of their ancestral homeland and its customs, traditions, and contributions can create a form of alienation from one's traditional cultural values and worldviews, a kind of cultural estrangement. More specifically, the racial inequality in access to wealth, education, cultural esteem, and social status associated with cultural oppression may place many African Americans at risk of compromising the overall vision of group advancement for personal gain (Schiele, 2005).

The civil rights and black power gains of the 1950s, 1960s, and 1970s have propelled greater numbers of African Americans into the middle and upper classes (Anderson, 2000; Billingsley, 1992; Franklin,

1997; Landry, 1987). As a result, there has been a growing underclass of African Americans who lack the training and skills needed to enter primary and legitimate labor markets (Anderson, 2000; Wilson, 1987, 1996). These parallel phenomena have created an increased class schism in the African-American community. The implication here is that the variation in social class status may lessen the psychoemotional bonds between African Americans who have more and African Americans who have less, which also may reduce the chances of preserving common cultural ties between the two.

Spiritual alienation is the last risk factor generated by cultural oppression. It is defined by Schiele (1996) as "the disconnection of nonmaterial and morally affirming values from concepts of human self-worth and from the character of social relationships" (p. 289). Cultural oppression is a primary source of the social problems experienced by African Americans and has placed them at risk of cultural estrangement, a weakened black collectivism, and spiritual alienation. Together, these risk factors make it difficult for African Americans, their communities, and their families to elicit their vast, positive human potentiality.

African Americans have undoubtedly demonstrated their resilience at overcoming the barriers of oppression, however, they continue to be exposed to Eurocentric cultural oppression (Schiele, 2005). This exposure may have diminished the spirit of collectiveness among African Americans and the desire to embrace cultural traditions, values, and practices.

WHAT THIS MEANS IN TODAY'S CONTEXT: THE IMPLICATIONS

Contemporary issues, our aging society, and the significance of multigenerational families require practitioners to be persistent in being creative. Though black kinship ties and self-reliance have been an effective tool of the past, today's unique conditions of a postindustrial society warrants a reinvention of these strings. A concerted effort of all systems, families, community organizations, and supportive groups within the African-American community is called for. Problems have become so severe and complex that ordinary citizens' kinship network, the African-American church, and grass roots organizations cannot tackle them alone. We must search for approaches that are deeply rooted in the African-American tradition, that have been effective in the past, and that can be reerected or revitalized to tackle the realties of the twenty-first century. Utilizing the power of intergenerational family and community ties, and strong kinship bonds makes sense and is a best practice and a good first step.

Embracing the legacies and wisdom of past generations and the hope and promise of the future provides a framework for best practices. This approach requires that family and community history, contemporary family and community life and resources are seen as multidimensional informants, resources, and assets.

This book presents content on African-American families and communities organized around an intergenerational perspective that recognizes transactions across generations. It incorporates the voices of African-American families and strengths-based teaching that prepares practitioners for competent practice with African-American families. Practice principles and the intergenerational perspective will provide a framework for exploring (1) the strength and resource richness of intergenerational relationships; (2) the roles and contributions of African-American elders, middle-aged adults, and children to family life; (3) the issues and challenges facing African-American multigenerational families and the extended family network; and (4) the impact of community intergenerational transactions. The authors discuss the intergenerational perspective and offer insight, program examples, and practice implementations.

REFERENCES

Anderson, E. (2000, March). The emerging Philadelphia African American class structure. *Annals of the American Academy of Political and Social Sciences, 568,* 54-75.

Bagley, C., & Carroll, J. (1998). Healing forces in African American families. In H. McCubbin, E. Thompson, A. Thompson, & J. Futrell (Eds.), *Resiliency in ethnic minority families.* Thousand Oaks, CA: Sage Publications.

The Balm In Gilead, Inc. (2007). Retrieved April 1, 2007 from http://www.balming ilead .org/about/mission.asp.

Barnes, S. L. (2001). Stressors and strengths: A theoretical and practical examination of nuclear, single-parent, and augmented African American families. *Families in Society: The Journal of Contemporary Human Services, 82*(5), 449-460.

Billingsley, A. (1992). *Climbing Jacob's ladder: The enduring legacy of African-American families.* New York: Simon & Schuster.

Billingsley, A. (1999). *Mighty like a river: The black church and social reform.* New York: Oxford University Press.

Billingsley, A., & Morrison-Rodriguez, B. (1998). The black family in the 21st century and the church as an action system: A macro perspective. *Journal of Human Behavior in the Social Environment, 1*(2-3), 31-47.

Boyd, T. (2004). *The new HNIC: Death of the civil rights and the reign of hip hop.* New York: NYU Press.

Boyd-Franklin, N. (1989). *Black families in therapy: A multisystems approach.* New York: Doubleday.

Boyd-Franklin (2003). *Black families in therapy: Understanding the African American experience.* New York: Guilford Press.

Byrd, W. M., & Clayton, L. A. (2000). *An American health dilemma: A medical history of African Americans and the problem of race: Beginnings to 1900.* New York: Routledge.

Carlton-LaNey, I. (2003). Stories from rural elderly African Americans. *Generations, 27*(3) fall, 34-38.

Carlton-LaNey, I. (2005). *African American aging in the rural South.* Durham, NC: Sourwood Press.

Cnaan, R. A., Boddie, S. C., & Kang, J. J. (2005). Religious congregations as social services providers for older adults. *Journal of Gerontological Social Work, 45*(1-2), 105-130.

Coyne-Beasley, T., & Schoenbach, V. J. (2000). The African-American church: A potential forum for adolescent comprehensive sexuality education. *Journal of Adolescent Health, 26*(4), 289-294.

Cox, C. B. (2002). Empowering African American custodial grandparents. *Social Work, 47*(1), 45-54.

Denby, R. W. (1996). Resiliency and the African American family: A model of family preservation. In S. Logan (Ed.), *The black family: Strengths, self help and positive change* (pp. 144-163). Boulder, CO: Westview Press.

Dunlap, E., Golub, A., & Johnson, B. D. (2006). The severely-distressed African American family in the crack era: Empowerment is not enough. *Journal of Sociology and Social Welfare, 33*(1), 115.

Dunlap, E., Golub, A., Johnson, B. D., & Wesley, D. (2002). Intergenerational transmission of conduct norms for drugs, sexual exploitation and violence: A case study. *British Journal of Criminology, 42,* 1-20.

Franklin, D. L. (1997). *Ensuring inequality: The structural transformation of the African American family.* New York: Oxford University Press.

Franklin, R. M. (2007). *Crisis in the village: Restoring hope in African American communities.* Minneapolis, MN: Fortress Press.

Freeman, E. M., & Logan, S. L. (Eds.) (2004). *Reconceptualizing the strengths and common heritage of black families.* Springfield, IL: Charles C Thomas

Gibson, P. A. (2005). Intergenerational parenting from the perspective of African American grandmothers. *Family Relations, 54*(2), 280.

Hill, R. (1972). *Strengths of the black family.* New York: Emerson Hall Publishers.

Hill, R. (1999). *The strengths of African American families: Twenty-five years later.* Lanham, MD: University Press of America.

Hines, P. M., & Boyd-Franklin, N. (1996). African American families. In M. McGoldrick, J. Giordano, & J. K. Peace (Eds.), *Ethnicity and family therapy* (pp. 66-84). New York: Guilford Press.

Hooyman, N., & Kiyak, H. A. (2005). *Social gerontology: A multidisciplinary perspective.* Needham Heights, MA: Allyn & Bacon.

Ladner, J. (1998). *The ties that bind: Timeless values for African American families.* Somerset, NJ: John Wiley.

Landry, B. (1987). *The new black middle class.* Berkeley, CA: University of California Press.

Lincoln, C. E., & Mamiya, L. H. (1990). *The black church in the African American experience.* Durham, NC: Duke University Press.

Logan, S. (2001). *The black family: Strengths, self help and positive change.* Boulder, CO: Westview Press.

McAdoo, A. P. (2002). *Diverse children of color: Research and policy implications.* In H. P. McAdoo (Ed.), *Black children* (2nd ed., pp. 13-26). Thousand Oaks, CA: Sage Publications.

McAdoo, H. (1997). *Black families.* Thousand Oaks, CA: Sage Publications.

McCubbin, H. (1998). *Resiliency in African-American families.* Thousand Oaks, CA: Sage Publications.

Min, J. W. (2005). Cultural competency: A key to effective future social work with racially and ethnically diverse elders. *Families in Society: The Journal of Contemporary Social Services, 86*(3), 347-358.

Morrison, J. D. (1991). The black church as a support system for black elderly. *Journal of Gerontological Social Work, 17*(1-2), 105-120.

Ruiz, D. S., & Carlton-LaNey, I. (1999). The increase in intergenerational African American families headed by grandmothers. *Journal of Sociology and Social Welfare, 26*(4), 71-86.

Saleebey, D. (1992). *The strengths perspective in social work practice.* White Plains, NY: Longman.

Scannapieco, M., & Jackson, S. (1996). Kinship care: The African American resilient response to family preservation. *Social Work, 41,* 190-196.

Schiele, J. H. (1996). Afrocentricity: An emerging paradigm in social work practice. *Social Work, 41*(3), 284-294.

Schiele, J. H. (2005). Cultural oppression and the high-risk status of African Americans. *Journal of Black Studies, 35*(6), 802-826.

Stack, C. B. (1996). *Call to home: African Americans reclaim the rural South.* New York: Basic Books.

Stack, C. B. (1997). *All our kin: Strategies for survival in a black community.* New York: Basic Books.

Staples, R. (1999). *The Black family: Essays and studies.* Belmont, CA: Wadsworth.

Sudarkasa, N. (1997). African American families and family values. In H. P. McAdoo (Ed.), *Black families* (3rd ed., pp. 9-40). Thousand Oaks, CA: Sage Publications.

Taylor, R. J., & Chatters, L. M. (1989). Families, friend, and church support networks of black Americans. In R. L Jones (Ed.), *Black adult development and aging.* Berkeley, CA: Cobb & Henry.

Taylor, R. J., Chatters, L. M., & Celious, A. K. (2003). Extended family households among black Americans. *African American Research Perspectives, 9,* 133-151.

Taylor, R. J., Jackson, J. S., & Chatters, L. M. (1997). *Family life in Black America.* Thousand Oaks, CA: Sage Press.

Walls, C. T., & Zarit, S. H. (1991). Informal support from black churches and the well-being of elderly blacks. *The Gerontologist, 31,* 490-495.

Wilson, W. J. (1987). *The truly disadvantaged: The inner city, the underclass, and public policy.* Chicago: University of Chicago.

Wilson, W. J. (1996). *When work disappears: The world of the new urban poor.* New York: Random House.

Chapter 2

Intergenerational Perspective

Cheryl Waites

If I don't care for you, I don't care for myself.

African proverb

One could say that a major strength of African Americans is the importance of the extended family, multigenerational units, and intergenerational relationships and transmissions. Without strong kinship bonds African-American families could not have survived the physical and psychic atrocities of slavery as well as the hardship of reconstruction, Jim Crow, and Depression eras. They would not have been able to come together and push the civil rights agenda forward and would not be advocating for a renewed commitment to the contemporary issues of drug, poverty, and the blatant economic and health disparities. Because of this legacy it's important to connect the past and present to move forward. This chapter describes an intergenerational model that can be used to understand and provide services to African-American families and communities. Using an approach that affords a look at family through family life cycle, life course, and generational lenses highlights the interconnectedness of African-American families, communities, and history. It allows us to look back and forward across time and generations.

DEMOGRAPHIC CHANGES:
POPULATION AGING

We are in the midst of a dramatic shift in the age distribution that directly impacts the probability of increased intergenerational

Social Work Practice with African-American Families

transactions. The population of older adults is expected to increase and transform the age structure in the United States. In 1900, the shape of the American population by age was that of a pyramid with a large base population band of children under age five (U.S. Bureau of the Census, 1996). By 2030, the age structure is predicted to look more like a rectangle with similar numbers in each category. More than 20 percent of Americans will be sixty-five or older. The number of African-American elders, aged sixty-five and older, is also growing. Between 1980 and 1995 there was an increase from 2.1 million to 2.7 million (a 29 percent increase). This group is expected to expand to 6.9 million by 2030 and 8.6 million by 2050 (Miles, 1999). This change in demographics will result in greater number of persons requiring health care, housing, nutrition assistance, caregiving, intergenerational programs, retirement communities, long-term care facilities, and other services. Over the next few decades all social workers can look forward to having experience working with older clients and their families (Kropf, 2002). In view of this transformation, social workers must be prepared to serve the needs of older adults and multigenerational families.

Individuals are now more likely to grow older in four- or even more generation families, spend an unprecedented number of years in family roles such as grandparenthood, and part of a more complex and varied web of intergenerational family ties (Bengtson, Rosenthal, & Burton, 1990; Hagestad, 1996; Hagestad & Neugarten, 1985; Riley, 1987). This demographic shift will impact all families. Perhaps African-American families and other ethnic and racial minorities, who have more collective and interdependent family networks, will lead the way in forging new family forms and intergenerational relationships. Attention to these intergenerational relationships calls for intergenerational approaches to address these issues and to empower families and communities to meet these challenges.

THEORETICAL UNDERPINNINGS OF AN INTERGENERATIONAL PERSPECTIVE

Intergenerational relationships describe multigenerational transactions by which persons of different generations interrelate with one another. The term intergenerational is most frequently used by practitioners and researchers and generally refers to relationships and interactions between two or more generations, most often the very young and the very old (see Kuehne, 1999; Rosenbrook & Larkin, 2002). At the societal level, relations among the generations are best embodied by the status of the social compact. This compact is an informal and unwritten "promise" between generations that "gives expression to and is based on the reciprocal ties that hold families, governance, and society together over time" (Cornman & Kingson, 1999, p. 10). The growing number of generations is also generating concerns about the efficient use of scarce resources among the generations and the potential for intergenerational conflict moved by inequality (Kingson & Williamson, 1993; Wisesale, 2003). These are issues that are moving to the forefront with the shift in demographics.

Bengtson (2001) suggests that family multigenerational relationships will be more important in the twenty-first century owing to (1) longer years of shared lives between generations; (2) the increasing importance of grandparents and other kin in fulfilling family functioning; and (3) the strength and resilience of intergenerational solidarity over time. It is also recognized that there is much diversity in intergenerational relationships because of changing family structure, increased longevity of kin, and other cultural and historical considerations.

There will be increasing availability of extended intergenerational kin (grandparents, great grandparents, uncles, and aunts) as resources for children as they move toward adulthood (Uhlemberg & Kirby, 1998; Wachter, 1997). Longer years of "shared lives" across generations are projected (Bengtson, 2001). More aging parents and grandparents will be available to provide family continuity and support across time (Silverstein, Giarrusso, & Bengtson, 1998). Networks of kin can be called upon to provide support for younger families (King, 1994; Silverstein, Parrott, & Bengtson, 1995) and to provide mentoring and guidance to emerging community leaders. These older kin may also be healthier than in past generations (Hayward & Heron, 1999), have greater access to preventive health care, and may be active well into old age.

Longer years of shared lives also bring more years of caregiving for dependent elders (Bengtson, Rosenthal, & Burton, 1990). In regard to relationships, lifelong trouble-ridden intergenerational relationships (i.e., parent-child relations) may produce continued conflict through the life course. The variety of family forms will also continue to be prevalent in the form of gay and lesbian families, single-parent families, childless families, grandparents (and in some cases great grandparents) raising grandchildren, and grandchildren caring for parents and grandparents. Intergenerational patterns of help and assistance flow mostly from the older generation to the younger generations in the family but can be reciprocal over time.

Intergenerational Solidarity

Bengtson and his colleagues (Bengtson & Roberts, 1991; Bengtson & Schrader, 1982) provide a comprehensive framework for understanding intergenerational relationships in later life. He argues that "multigenerational bonds are more important than nuclear family ties for well-being and support over the life course" (Bengtson, 2001, p. 7). Within their intergenerational solidarity framework, behavioral and emotional dimensions are examined that address effectual, associated, consensual functional normative, and structural solidarity (see Table 2.1). These five domains provide a framework for understanding intergenerational relationships.

TABLE 2.1. Intergenerational Practice Model

Domain	Issues to Assess and Address	Strengths to Build or Empower
Affectional Solidarity Expressed sentiment about relationships. How much affection do family members share. Generational ties	• Traditions regarding intergenerational ties, sentiment, and relationships • Intergenerational emotional ties and obligation • Filial crisis inter-generational conflict • Affiliations and ties with community	• Life course and family life cycle understanding • Relationship building across generations • Cultural knowledge, traditions, and pride— consciousness raising
Associational Solidarity Type and frequency of contact between generations	• Intergenerational family dynamics and transac-tions • Access to intergenerational family	• Communication networks • Family reunions, celebrations, and intergenerational events

Domain	Issues to Assess and Address	Strengths to Build or Empower
	• members, community programs, and activities • Literacy and technology literacy	• Cross-generations information sharing and support
Consensual Solidarity Agreement in opinions, values, and orientation between generations	• Generational values differences • Generational values similarities • Generation gap	• Shared history and values • Recognition of each generation's unique strengths • Intergenerational respect • Shared visions
Functional Solidarity Giving and receiving support across generations	• Help-seeking and help-receiving behavior and traditions • Role of the church and informal institutions • Role of formal institutions • Individualism versus collectivism orientations	• Flexible family roles • Equable care • Utilization of informal and formal support system • Healthy lifestyle
Normative Solidarity Expectations regarding filial obligation and parental and community obligation	• Filial responsibilities— for example, intergenerational support for at-risk youth, young families, and dependent elders • Older and middle generation obligations • Parenting traditions • Mentoring traditions	• Afrocentric perspective— the village concept (it takes a village) • Variety of caregiving roles • Integration support, mentoring, and civic engagement
Structural Solidarity Opportunity for cross-generational interaction reflecting geographic proximity	• Migration patterns • Housing and coresidence issues • Possible locations to facilitate cross-generational connections • Transportation and travel distances	• Collaboration and support across generations • Intergenerational programming • Intergenerational interdependence • Public policy that recognizes and addresses the needs of all generations • Community intergenerational activities • Local community unit(s) that promote intergenerational relationships

Source: Adapted from Bengtson and Roberts, 1991, Intergenerational Solidarity Model.

As we look to extended years of shared lives, the dynamics of inter-generational exchanges will have a variety of implications for families. Some may experience a clash in values between the traditional family ideals of an older generation and the values adopted by their children and grandchildren. Conversely, many years of shared lives may bring together families' strengths, resilience, and solidarity. It will be important for practitioners to understand these issues, utilize skills, and develop resources that help families navigate these complex and changing relationships. To this end, other theoretical frameworks can inform this process.

Life Course

The life course perspective is a tool for understanding the dynamics of relationships and identity formation in context and over time (Bengtson & Allen, 1993; Elder, 1985, 1998). Life course theory emerged in the 1960s out of the need to understand human development as occurring across the life span. Elder has been a pioneer in this field that emphasizes how individual lives are socially patterned over time and the processes by which lives are changed by changing environments. Age-graded life course describes the time of life and the place or context. The life course is age graded through institutions and social structures, and it is embedded in relationships that constrain and support behavior. "Both the individual life course and a person's developmental trajectory are interconnected with the lives and development of others" (Elder, 1998, pp. 951-952). The life course perspective offers four concepts—human agency, linked lives, location in context, and multiple rhythms of time (Giele & Elder, 1998; Patton, 2002).

Agency refers to how individuals construct their own life course through the choices they make and actions they take within the opportunities and constraints of history and social circumstances (Elder, 1985), while *linked lives* refer to how lives are lived interdependently, and social and historical influences are expressed through a network of shared relationships. *Location in context* informs us that diverse social context provides insight into family networks across generations. New generation emerged into different social and economic realities than previous generations. For example, those born during the hip-hop generation have a different connection with the Civil Rights

Movement than those who lived through it. The *multiple rhythms in time* weave three concepts together through the interplay of multiple time perspectives. First, timing in lives—the individual time and the developmental impact of life transitions or events. Next there is generational time—moving to the next developmental stage with your age cohort, connecting with another generations, and building within family and extended family relationships. Then there is time and place—the sociohistorical events that shape the cohort experiences. For example, the events surrounding 9/11 will forever shape all generational cohorts relative to developmental stage and generational time (World War II veterans, versus Baby Boomers, versus Generation X). The life course of individuals are embedded in and shaped by the historical times and places they experience over their lifetime.

Family Life Cycle

Families are made of people who have shared history and future (Carter & McGoldrick, 1999). They are the natural context within which individual development takes place. A family as it moves through times together is often referred to as family life cycle stages. Relationships with parents, siblings, and other family members go through transitions as they move along the life cycle. Theses stages have been identified as leaving home, single young adults, joining of families through marriage, the new couple, and families with young children, families with adolescents, launching children and moving on, and families in later life (Carter & McGoldrick, 1999).

There is much variety in family forms, and diversity in structure and function is evident in African-American families. Single-parent families (mother or father) may or may not establish parental and grandparental relationships after children are born. Alternately, extended family may play a more important role in family support and care. Grandparents may step in to assist or raise grandchildren. These are just a few variations, yet it is recognized that with some diversity in structure and function families pass through stages. These stages are impacted by the era of history that the family is embedded in, as well as the agency, lived lives, location, and the multiple rhythms in time of its members.

Individuals develop in the context of families and the larger social context with past and present properties. Each system has properties that change over time. Carter and McGoldrick (1999) describe the two-dimensional, horizontal, and vertical flow of stress in family life. The vertical flow brings past and present on all levels and the horizontal that is developmental and unfolding. The vertical influences are the biological heritage, temperament, and genetic makeup (Carter & McGoldrick, 1999). It also includes family history, the patterns of relating and functioning that are transmitted down the generations, and historical events such as the political climate, war, and so on. The horizontal relates to the emotional, cognitive, interpersonal, and physical development over the life span within a historical context. It describes the family as it moves through time, coping with changes and transitions in the family life cycle, as well as the community context and societal conditions such as racism, sexism, classism, ageism, and so on. Intergenerational relationships with parents, siblings, and extended family members go through transitions as they move along the life cycle. The community and environmental realities add dimension and context. Cultural, historical, and social factors also shape individuals, families, and communities.

Afrocentric Paradigm

An Afrocentric perspective focuses on traditional African philosophical assumptions, which emphasize holistic, interdependent, and spiritual conception of people and their environment (Schiele, 2000). It affirms that there are universal cultural strengths of an African worldview that survived the generational devastations caused by the transatlantic slave trade and the oppression that followed. It also recognizes that diversity exists among Africans and those of African descent and expresses the utility of African-centered value-based practices. These practices integrate cultural strengths into micro, mezzo, and macro interventions used to enhance the lives of all people but particularly people of color. An Afrocentric paradigm fits nicely with the intergenerational perspective because it affirms human capabilities, family and cultural strengths, and promotes intergenerational connections.

Cultural Competence and Humility

The intergenerational perspective is compatible with culturally competent practice. Culturally competent practice has been described as the ability to effectively apply social work skills in a way that is knowledgeable and respectful of a client's culture (Weaver, 1999). Cultural competence involves providing services that are perceived as legitimate for addressing problems experienced by culturally diverse people (Crewe, 2004; Green, 1999). It denotes the ability to transform knowledge and cultural awareness into interventions that support and sustain healthy client-system functioning (McPhatter, 1997). When working with African-American families and communities, it is important to acknowledge traditions, worldviews, and strengths of cultural groups while remaining open to the dynamic nature of culture (Waites, Macgowan, Pennell, Carlton-LaNey, & Weil, 2004). In regard to African Americans, cultural competence is enhanced when intergenerational relationships and multigenerational families and communities are delineated and understood.

To achieve some form of cultural competence one might practice cultural humility. This is an approach used in health fields and has been described by Tervalon and Murray-Garcia (1998) as a lifelong process of self-reflection and self-critique. The provider/practitioner is encouraged to develop a respectful partnership with each client through client-focused interviewing, exploring similarities and differences between his own and each patient's priorities, goals, and capacities.

WHAT IS INTERGENERATIONAL PRACTICE?

Intergenerational relationships describe multigenerational transactions by which persons of different age cohorts interrelate with one another. Intergenerational practice reflects a framework that brings an awareness and attention to these relationships. It builds on the life course and family life cycle models, and recognizes the family as a system moving through time (Carter & McGoldrick, 1999). It is a method by which one can understand how generations provide mutual support to each other during times of need and seek to both contribute and create better futures for successive generations (Cornman & Kingson, 1999). This approach also brings an Afrocentric perspective to enhance cultural understanding and places importance on a holistic viewpoint.

The intergenerational practice perspective expands on the family life cycle model and acknowledges the interconnectedness of family, extended family, and community. It reflects an approach to work with families and communities that respects and supports the strengths and resilience of intergenerational solidarity over time while acknowledging issues that may arise. Intergenerational practice is a perspective whose basic principles promote a society that values all generations as well as

- recognizes that each generation has unique strengths, each person, young and older, is a resource;
- recognizes the roles of youths and elders in families and communities;
- acknowledges conflicts that may occur in intergenerational transactions;
- encourages collaboration and support across generations;
- fosters intergenerational interdependence; and
- fosters public policy that recognizes and addresses the needs of all generations.

The intergenerational perspective supports family and extended family members interacting across their life course in providing assistance and care. It highlights communities and organizations comprising multigenerations working together to address community needs through intergenerational cooperation and partnerships. Intergenerational practice reflects a perspective that respects and supports these relationships and brings together resources that connect the generations. An intergenerational practice model that may be used with African-American families is described in Table 2.1. This model includes six domains adapted from Bengtson and his colleagues' (Bengtson & Roberts, 1991; Bengtson & Schrader, 1982) intergenerational solidarity framework, for understanding intergenerational relationships in later life.

An Intergenerational Practice Model

An intergenerational approach considers generational transmission from a strengths perspective, looking not only at problems passed down through the generations but also the assets that successive generations provide and that can be drawn from. It is a framework that helps extract power, resilience, and capital from past and current relationships and traditions. There are six domains that are linked to issues to assess and strengths to build or empower.

The first domain, *affectional solidarity* (see Table 2.1), addresses the expressed sentiment regarding intergenerational relationships. It calls for the practitioner to look at emotional ties to family and community, intergenerational conflict, as well as the overall affiliation with the ethnic/racial cultural group (or community/cultural context). The goal is to assess and address the issues and build on the strengths, and to empower relational understanding and cultural knowledge across the life course or family life cycle. The second domain, *associational solidarity,* focuses on the type and frequency of contact between generations. Assessing intergenerational communication dynamics and interactions informs this domain and can lead to improved communication networks, and enhance the amount and quality of intergenerational contact. Often enhancing one's ability to utilize technology effectively can be beneficial, especially to older adults who may not be technologically literate and have limited access to or competence in using cell phones or e-mail. The third domain, *consensual solidarity,* looks at agreements of values and opinion. Here the generation gap is explored and the mechanism to build intergenerational respect, dialogue, shared vision, and collaboration are of importance. The fourth domain, *functional solidarity,* looks at giving and receiving support across generations. The roles that individualism and collectivism play in help-seeking and help-giving behaviors as well as the significance of informal and formal support systems are assessed. Mechanisms to enhance equable intergenerational care and the use of formal and informal resources and institutions are implemented. The fifth domain, *normative solidarity,* looks at filial responsibility and traditions. Using Afrocentric traditions, while remaining flexible to the diversity of situations, and building informal and formal resources through mentoring, community programs and civic engagement, are stressed. The sixth domain, *structural solidarity,* highlights the opportunities for intergenerational interaction as it relates to proximity. Some older adults reside with their children or grandchildren in coresidential situations. However, migration patterns of younger adults' families as well as transportation issues impact opportunities to maintain close contacts. Often older adults are unable to travel to family or community events due to distant locations or limited access to convenient and affordable transportation.

Social workers can use the intergenerational practice model for understanding and working with individuals and families, communities, and for advocacy and policy practice. This model can be instrumental in addressing intergenerational issues that are moving to the forefront as our society ages.

Intergenerational Issues

There are several relevant intergenerational issues that families face—kinship care, grandparents raising grandchildren, the "boomerang" generation (young adults who return home), caring for dependent elders, caregiver health and support, guardianship and other legal issues, intergenerational values transmission, as well as health and well-being. Multigenerational kin and extended family networks are all relevant to this perspective.

These issues are also relevant to communities. Children, younger adults, and elders benefit from intergenerational partnerships that lead to stronger communities. Affordable housing, health care and health disparities, formal child care and elder care, education for youths and continuing education for adults, recreation and leisure activities, prevention programs, for example, nutrition, exercise, friendly visiting, mentoring, tutoring, educational enrichment, and job training are community programs that serve to preserve and strengthen families and communities.

Intergenerational policy and formal programs must address the increased number of multigenerational families and communities. Elders are community assets and a source for community leadership and civic engagement. They can and they do serve as volunteers, teachers, and mentors. With improved health, increased longevity, early retirement, and time to devote to community pursuits, older adults have and will continue to have the opportunity to retain their roles as productive members of their community. A policy that is intergenerational promotes the interdependence of the generations, views people of all ages as resources, is sensitive to intergenerational family structures and diverse family forms, and encourages intergenerational transfers through shared care or services. As society ages, policy and programs will need to efficiently address intergenerational issues and design effective ways to meet the needs of multigenerations.

IMPLICATIONS

Adopting an intergenerational framework provides a mechanism to address or facilitate (1) intergenerational partnerships; (2) intergenerational exchanges and the contribution of elders; and (3) opportunities for transactions across generations, encouraging intergenerational policy and programs that nurture and support families, communities, and organizations. As we move through this century this model may prove to be very relevant to the changing demographics of our aging society.

REFERENCES

Bengtson, V. L. (2001). Beyond the nuclear family: The increasing importance of multigenerational relationships in American society. 1998 Burgess Award Lecture. *Journal of Marriage and the Family, 63*(1), 1-16.

Bengtson, V. L., & Allen, K., R., (1993). The life course perspective applied to families over time. In R. Boss, W. Doherty, R. LaRossa, W. Schumm, & S. Steinmetz (Eds.), *Sourcebook of family theories and methods: A contextual approach* (pp. 469-498). New York: Plenum Press.

Bengtson, V. L., & Roberts, R. E. L. (1991). Intergenerational solidarity in aging families: An example of formal theory construction. *Journal of Marriage and the Family, 53,* 856-870.

Bengtson, V. L., Rosenthal, C. J., & Burton, L. M., (1990). Paradoxes of families and aging. In R. H. Binstock & L. K. George (Eds.), *Handbook of aging and the social sciences* (4th ed., pp. 253-282). San Diego, CA: Academic Press.

Bengtson, V. L., & Schrader, S. S. (1982). Parent-child relations. In D. Mangen & W. Peterson (Eds.), *Handbook of research instruments in social gerontology* (vol. 2, pp. 115-185). Minneapolis, MN: University of Minnesota press.

Carter, B., & McGoldrick, M. (1999). *The expanded family life* (3rd ed.). Boston, MA: Allyn & Bacon.

Cornman, J. M., & Kingson, E. R. (Winter 1999). Yes, John, there is a social compact. *Generations, 22*(4), 10-14.

Crewe, S. (2004). Ethnogerontology: Preparing culturally competent social workers for the diverse facing of aging. *Journal of Gerontological Social Work, 43*(4), 45-58.

Elder, G. H. Jr. (1985). *Life course dynamics.* Ithaca, NY: Cornell University Press.

Elder, G. H. Jr. (1998). The life course as developmental theory. *Child Development, 69,* 1-12.

Giele, J. Z., & Elder, G. H. Jr. (1998). *Methods of life course research: Qualitative and quantitative approaches.* Thousand Oaks, CA: Sage Publications.

Green, J. (1999). *Cultural awareness in the human services* (3rd ed.). Boston, MA: Allyn & Bacon.

Hagestad, G. O. (1996). On-time, off-time, out of time? Reflections on continuity and discontinuity from an illness process. In V. L. Bengtson (Ed.), *Adulthood and aging: Research on continuities and discontinuities* (pp. 204-222). New York: Springer.

Hagestad, G. O., & Neugarten, B. L. (1985). Age and the life course. In R. H. Binstock & E. Shanas (Eds.), *Handbook of aging and the social sciences.* New York: Van Nostrand Reinhold.

Hayward, M., & Heron, M. (1999). Racial inequality in active life among adult Americans. *Demography, 36*(1), 77-91.

King, V. (1994). Variation in the consequences of non-resident father involvement for children's well-being. *Journal of Marriage & Family, 56,* 963-972.

Kingson, E. R., & Williamson, J. B. (1993). The generational equity debate. A progressive framing of a conservative issue. *Journal of Aging and Social Policy, 5,* 31-53.

Kropf, N. (2002). Strategies to increase student interest in aging. *Journal of Gerontological Social Work, 39*(1/2), 57-67.

Kuehne, V. S. (1999). Building intergenerational communities through research and evaluation. *Generations, 22*(4), 82-87.

McPhatter, A. R. (1997). Cultural competence in child welfare: What is it? How do we achieve it? What happens without it? *Child Welfare, 76,* 255-278.

Miles, T. P. (1999). *Living with chronic disease and the policies that bind.* In T. P. Miles (Ed.), *Full-color aging: Facts, goals, and recommendations for America's diverse elders* (pp. 53-63). Washington, DC: Gerontological Society of America.

Patton, M. Q. (2002). *Qualitative research and evaluation methods* (3rd ed.). Thousand Oaks, CA: Sage Publications.

Riley, M. W. (1987). On the significance of age in sociology. *American Sociological Review, 52,* 1-14.

Rosenbrook, V., & Larkin, E. (2002). Introducing standards and guidelines: A rationale for defining the knowledge, skills and dispositions of intergenerational practice. *Journal of Intergenerational Relationships, 1,* 133-144.

Schiele, J. H. (2000). *Human services and the Afrocentric paradigm.* Binghamton, NY: The Haworth Press.

Silverstein, M., Giarrusso, R., & Bengtson, V. (1998). Intergenerational solidarity and the grandparent role. In M. Szinovacz (Ed.), *The handbook on grandparenthood.* Westport, CT: Greenwood Press.

Silverstein, M., Parrott, T. M., & Bengtson, V. L. (1995). Factors that predispose middle-aged sons and daughters to provide social support to older parents. *Journal of Marriage and the Family, 57*(2), 465-475.

Tervalon, M., & Murray-Garcia, J. (1998). Cultural humility versus cultural competence: A critical distinction in defining physician training outcomes. *Journal of Health Care for the Poor and Underserved, 99,* 2.

Uhlenberg, P., & Kirby, J. B. (1998). Grandparenthood over time: Historical and demographic trends. In M. E. Szinovacz (Ed.), *Handbook on grandparenthood* (pp. 23-39). Westport, CT: Greenwood Press.

U.S. Census Bureau (1996). Current population reports. Retrieved November 20, 2006 from http://www.census.gov/prod/1/pop/p25-1130/.

Wachter, K. W. (1997). Kinship resources for the elderly. *Philosophical Transactions of the Royal Society of London B, 352*(1363), 1811-1817.

Waites, C., Macgowan, M., Pennell, J., Carlton-LaNey, I., & Weil, M. (2004). Increasing the cultural responsiveness of family group conferencing. *Social Work, 49,* 291-301.

Weaver, H. N. (1999). Indigenous people and the social work profession: Defining culturally competent services. *Social Work, 44*(3), 217-225.

Wisesale, S. K. (2003). Global aging and intergenerational equity. *Journal of Intergenerational Relationships, 1,* 29-47.

PART II:
INTERGENERATIONAL PRACTICE AND PROGRAMS

This section will discuss the intergenerational perspective and offer insight, program examples, and practice implementations.

Chapter 3

Genograms
with African-American Families:
Considering Cultural Context[*]

Annie McCullough-Chavis
Cheryl Waites

The family genogram is one of the most practical and widely accepted tools used in family therapy (Goldenberg & Goldenberg, 2000; Hartman, 1995; Hartman & Laird, 1983; McGoldrick & Gerson, 1985; McGoldrick, Gerson, & Shellenberger, 1999). It is extremely valuable for gathering information about families (Beck 1987; Guerin & Pendagast, 1976; Hartman & Laird, 1983; Kilpatrick & Holland, 2003; McGoldrick, Gerson, & Shellenberger, 1999) and can be especially useful when working with families from diverse backgrounds (Bean, Perry, & Bedell, 2002; Congress, 1994; Thomas, 1998). Social workers often work with families who are members of a variety of cultural and ethnic groups. In this regard, social workers and other practitioners are encouraged to become culturally competent (Green, 1999; Lum, 2000; Sowers & Ellis, 2001). Cultural competence requires an understanding of the traditions, worldviews, and strengths of cultural groups while remaining open to the dynamic nature of culture (Waites, Macgowan, Pennell, Carlton-LaNey, & Weil, 2004). For work with African Americans, this requires an understanding of the dimensions of African-American family life and cultural context. Resources such as strong kinship bonds, role flexibility, strong religious orientation, and strong

Previously published in *Journal of Family Social Work* 8(2), 2004. © 2004 by The Haworth Press, Inc. All rights reserved.

Social Work Practice with African-American Families

education/work ethic (Alston & Turner, 1994; Hill, 1997), as well as extended family networks and transactions must be considered when working with African-American families. Tools that enable practitioners to gain a better understanding and identify relevant resources or strengths are indicated.

The genogram provides an excellent means to illustrate the family systems process (McGoldrick, 1995). With some enrichment, the genogram can reflect significant cultural influences. This chapter presents an approach to completing genograms with African-American families. We have adapted the genogram so that it reveals family drama—family issues and transactions—as well as the broader cultural context. Intergenerational history, values, principles, traditions, and solidarity are addressed.

GENOGRAMS: CAPTURING FAMILY HISTORY AND CULTURAL CONTEXT

How Genograms Are Used

The genograms are a pictorial representation of a family used to help the practitioner understand the family situation and to increase self- and family awareness (Bahr, 1990). It typically expands across three or more generations and focuses on intergenerational patterns and relationships among family members. This visual tool can be used to trace family influences in various contexts as well as in the broader system (McGoldrick & Gerson, 1985). Genograms emphasize family dynamics but also can facilitate understanding individuals and families within a life cycle framework that is culturally relevant. The cultural context is an important aspect of the family's story and plays a significant role in family development. Adding cultural context to the standard model produces a cultural genogram (CG) that maps a family's race, ethnicity, migration history, religious history, social class, and cultural characteristics (Congress, 1994; Hardy & Laszloffy, 1995; McGoldrick, Giordano, & Pearce, 1996).

Cultural genograms have been used for rapport building, assessment, and as a mechanism for culturally competent practice. CGs, which build upon the basic genogram construction, have been suggested as a tool to enable practitioners to understand aspects of culture for families that have immigrated to the United States (Congress, 1994). Assessing the impact of culture on the family and individual is emphasized. Estrada and Haney (1998) and Thomas (1998) demonstrate with case examples how to use genograms to assess a multicultural context and establish rapport with diverse families. DeMaria, Weeks, and Hof (1999) and Hardy and Laszloffy (1995) used CG to enhance the understanding of culture and ethnicity in the lives of therapists and clients. Many have since used CGs as a training tool to enhance family therapists' awareness, sensitivity to diversity, and to encourage cultural competence (Bean et al., 2002; Hardy & Laszloffy, 1992, 1995; Keiley et al., 2002).

Genograms have also been augmented to highlight specific influences that impact family values, beliefs, traditions, and practices. Spiritually focused genograms are suggested as a potential vehicle for gaining an in-depth understanding of the spiritual dimensions and resources of clients (Dunn & Dawes, 1999; Frame, 2000; Hodge, 2001). Spirituality is a fundamental dimension that shapes one's perspective, particularly among African Americans, Hispanics, women, and older adults (Gallup & Lindsay, 1999). Spiritual genograms are used to provide a graphic representation of complex expressions of spirituality over three generations for assessment and intervention (Dunn & Dawes, 1999; Hodge, 2001).

Magnuson and Norem (1995) illustrate how genogram construction can be incorporated in the therapeutic process with gay and lesbian clients. They suggest that exploring the past family relationship patterns can help gay and lesbian clients develop "increased levels of self-differentiation and enhance their overall mental health in a nonaccepting society that engenders shame, fear, guilt, depression, loneliness and anxiety in gay men and lesbians" (Magnuson & Norem, 1995, p. 111). White and Tyson-Rawson (1995) utilized genograms to assess gender dynamics in couples and families.

Clearly, genograms have been used with diverse families to explore diverse aspects of family, social, and cultural influences. The literature indicates that using genograms that include a cultural focus—incorporating family history and the broader cultural context—can be useful.

Cultural Context

The broader cultural context refers to the environment and cultural influences. It recognizes that society, community, as well as cultural heritage, values, beliefs, thinking, and traditions impact families. Over-generalization of specific cultural groups moves practitioners away from culturally competent practice and does not recognize within group diversity, which is not our intent. Our framework for understanding culture and the cultural context is to recognize it as a transactional and a negotiated process rather than a cluster of qualities (Barth, 1969; Bennett, 1975). The ways in which that distinctiveness is defended, asserted, preserved, or abandoned amount to ethnic or cultural identity (Green, 1982). Culture is a mingling of traditions, values, religious beliefs, worldviews, thinking, and patterns of social interaction (Lum, 2000; Waites et al., 2004). The cultural context comprises the "boundaries that groups define around themselves, using selected cultural traits as criteria or markers of exclusion or inclusion" (Green, 1982, p. 12).

Culture includes the consideration of oppression, racism, harsh social conditions, as well as sources of resilience, strength, and intergenerational interdependence (Billingsley, 1992; Hill, 1997; Nobles, 1997; McAdoo, 1997). The practitioner's role is to use the CG to explore with the client, their cultural context. Once a therapist has established an alliance of trust with the family, Hines and Boyd-Franklin (1996) point out, genograms can be useful for gathering information on complex family systems in African-American families. This information can encourage, assist, enable, support, stimulate, and unleash the strengths within families and individuals, and empower or help them help themselves (Cowger, 1994).

AFRICAN-AMERICAN FAMILIES

A Historical Glimpse

Understanding African-American families requires an appreciation of the unique realities that have shaped their experience. Prevalent within the African-American broader cultural context is a connection to the past. "The African American family is not simply a functional adaptation to new social conditions, but a product of history and culture that has been conducive to the survival of the African American family" (McDaniel, 1990, p. 7). In spite of the harsh oppression and pervasive separation from their cultural heritage, traditions, and original languages, some African cultural expressions remain intact. Values connected with spirituality, special care for children, kinship ties, unity, and security have roots in the African past (Barnes, 2001; Nobles, 1974, 1991). Through cultural resilience, much of this heritage has evolved into many of the strengths of contemporary African-American families' systems in America.

Contemporary Strengths and Characteristics in African-American Families

Commonly recognized strengths in African-American families include the following:

1. Flexibility in family roles accompanied by strong intergenerational ties (Hill, 1997).
2. Emphasis on extended kinship network where family members and fictive kin are linked in terms of obligation and support (Hill, 1997).
3. Caregiving—special care for children and elders—primacy is given to children and elders are respected and revered (Billingsley, 1992; Sudarkasa, 1997).
4. Reciprocity, a sense of interdependence, feelings of "oneness" (Hall & King, 1982; Pinderhughes, 1982), or family solidarity.
5. The fundamental nature of spirituality and prominent role of religion (Billingsley, 1992, 1999; Boyd-Franklin, 1989; Dunn & Dawes, 1999; Hill, 1997).

Hill (1997) refers to the importance of the African-derived cultural strength of flexibility of family roles, where relationships and role functions between men and women are ideally egalitarian. Parenting is often a shared responsibility, and children may perform some parental functions for younger siblings. The extended kinship network often includes biological kin and fictive kin who provide emotional, social, and financial support such as advising, parenting, childcare, and informal adoptions (Boyd-Franklin, 1989; Hill, 1997; Lum, 2000). Adult members have a collective social, financial, and ethical responsibility to care for family members. Often family members will step in for absent parents or care for aging relatives. This network also socializes children to adapt to the dominant culture and helps them to cope with the realities of racism and oppression. When functioning at an optimal level the extended family support network helps family members adapt and survive throughout the life cycle.

The orientation where family takes precedence over the individual is well documented (Billingsley, 1992; Hill, 1997; Hines & Boyd-Franklin, 1996). Boyd-Franklin (1989) concludes that reciprocity, the process of helping each other, and exchanging and sharing support as well as goods and services, is a central part of the lives of African Americans. This principle compels one to give back to their family and community in return for what had been given to them (Sudarkasa, 1997). African Americans place a high premium on mutual assistance and interdependence; it remains an important value (Billingsley, 1999; Hill, 1997). This is evident in the prevalence of the extended family network where several households are centered on a base unit (Burton, 2003; Martin & Martin, 1978). Owing to migration, the network and base household may span several communities or states but remain significant. The base household is usually the home of the family's recognized leader. These family leaders influence the affairs, traditions, and practices of the entire extended network. They are often the glue that binds the family together and reinforces a strong expectation for cooperation and reciprocity.

Grandparents, and particularly grandmothers, play a central role in African-American extended families (Billingsley, 1992, 1999). They serve as guardians and caretakers for their children, grandchildren, parents, many extended family members, and fictive kin. Grandparents represent wisdom and strength and are the keepers of family values such as respect, religion, love, support, and community. Grandparents, and especially grandmothers, are serving more frequently as surrogate parents owing to an increase in single and adolescent parenting, divorce, crime, HIV/AIDS, and drug usage (Barnes, 2001; Ruiz & Carlton-LaNey, 1999) and this has created stress on this valued resource. Often these middle-aged adults are responsible for several generations, including their children, nieces and nephews, as well as parents and other elder family members (Ruiz & Carlton-LaNey, 1999).

Spiritual and religious practices are a major resource for African-American families (Hines & Boyd-Franklin, 1996; Pipes, 1997). African

Americans are known to be spiritual people (Sudarkasa, 1997). Spirituality and religion are generally understood to be distinct, but overlapping (Carroll, 1998; Pellebon & Anderson, 1999). Spirituality is defined as an invisible material that connects all human beings to one another and to the Creator (Schiele, 2000). It is a belief in the sacredness and interconnectedness of all life manifested in a quest for goodness and certain values. Religion is the formal institution that provides for the expression of spiritual beliefs and practices. Religion or religious belief is defined as the aspects of spirituality that are in the context of a formalized religious framework like the church (Dunn & Dawes, 1999). It is the adherence to the prescribed rituals, beliefs, and practices associated with the worship of God or a higher power.

Religion flows from spirituality; spirituality is often manifested in the form of association with an organized religious institution, like the church. Many African Americans have been reared with a belief in God or a higher power and the black church is the primary means in which many express their religious and spiritual beliefs and values (Billingsley, 1999; Hines & Boyd-Franklin, 1996; Richardson & June, 1997). Churches, and other religious institutions (i.e., mosques) prevalent in the African-American community provide a spiritual foundation; furthermore, religion is linked to cultural epistemology and offers a context for living. Religious institutions provide a moral voice that permits one to confront existential concerns and engage in self-reflection; offer coping resources and a means of dealing with adversity; and make available concrete services that function to preserve families. Religion and spiritual beliefs provide a foundation of inner strength and continue to be important in the lives of African-American families (Barnes, 2001).

Challenges and the Practitioner's Role

As three or more generations adjust to life-cycle transitions, these contemporary strengths or characteristics, when in place, provide assistance and care, and mitigate the often-difficult realities for African-American families. When contending with harsh social issues, specifically drug use, unemployment, poverty, less than adequate education, and inadequate housing, it is important to recognize strengths and other values that might help rescue families (Sudarkasa, 1997). Many families are overburdened by troubled circumstances, are overwhelmed with problems, or feel ashamed for having difficulties. This often makes it difficult for them, and others, to see their abilities and resources. Feelings of embarrassment, as well as the prevalence of racism, can prevent many African Americans from being able to appreciate their individual successes and/or the strengths and resources within their ethnic heritage and community. A focus on heritage reminding in the form of examining past problem solving and relating it to current problems (Manns, 1981) may be beneficial. This process requires cultural exploration and cultural knowledge, which the CG can facilitate. In addition, examining social supports and other strengths to handle negative environmental constraints may serve to empower clients.

The role of the social worker is to understand families and contemporary characteristics, to illuminate the strengths in their families and their broader social/cultural context, and to support families in taking control of their situation. CG promotes this process. It combines the standard genogram focus of understanding intergenerational patterns and history with an exploration of cultural heritage, influences, and strengths and resources.

THE CULTURAL GENOGRAM
WITH AFRICAN-AMERICAN FAMILIES

The CG used with African-American families takes into account cultural heritage and influences as well as intergenerational family values, patterns, transactions, and strengths. Building on the identified contemporary strengths and characteristics of African-American families, five areas and several key questions are identified to assist practitioners in gathering information for the CG. The five areas are as follows:

1. role flexibility;
2. extended family networks;
3. caregiving—special care for children and elders, impaired family members, and giving back to the community;
4. spirituality and religious beliefs and practices; and
5. family history, beliefs, values, rituals, and traditions (see Table 3.1).

TABLE 3.1. Cultural Context

Areas to Consider	Possible Cultural Influences	Family's Cultural Influences and Context
Role flexibility, family roles	• Role flexibility • Family leaders • Intergenerational relationships of ties	• Siblings sharing caretaking duties • Leadership in transition • Sibling caring for father and grandchild at home
Extended family networks	• Network of blood relatives and fictive kin • Other social support system • Reciprocity—obligation to family • Shared resources	• Strong family bond • Church, club, and sorority • Family pulling together for father's care at home • Financial and emotional support given despite the health and career issues of Nia and siblings
Caregiving—special care	• Primacy of children • Respect and care for the elders • Care for impaired relatives and ficitive kin • Reciprocity—giving back to family and community	• Family share responsibility • Father's wish is respected • Strong belief in caring for relatives and others • Active participation in church and community
Spirituality and religious beliefs and practices	• What is the meaning of spiritual and religious beliefs • Level of involvement in religious institutions • Participation in religious sponsored activity • Role of religion in every day life • Use of prayer and other religious practices	• Faith and a strong belief in a higher being • Active members and church leaders • Active in church activities • Daily Bible reading and praying • Pray in times of stress and joy, family prayer circle for all events
Family history, beliefs, rituals, and traditions	• Intergenerational family history, myths, customs, and practices • Family events, celebrations, and traditions • Education and achievement • Work ethics and employment • Meaning of illnesses and genetic predisposition • Physical and mental health access and practices	• Based leader (elder) • Graduations, birthdays, family reunions, and holidays celebrated at leader's house • College degrees expected • Hard workers and leaders • Live with illnesses unless God stops you • Hospice and medical care, pastoral and family advice

The CG reveals family traditions that are often mechanisms that promote family solidarity and strength. A sense of reciprocity permeates all five areas; it is infused in family roles, networks, caregiving, traditions, and spirituality.

The questions listed as follows help practitioners obtain pertinent information and insights around family history, transactions, and cultural context. In the list, a primary question is suggested and numbered. Follow-up questions are included to help practitioners and clients explore each of the five areas.

Questions

1. What is the makeup of your family?
   - Who lives in your household?
   - Whom do you include in your extended family network?
   - What are the roles of adult members?
2. How are elders viewed in your family?
   - What role do elders play in your family?
   - Who are considered the recognized leaders in your family?
   - Who are the family members you admire? Please explain.
   - How is caregiving to elders handled in your family?
3. How are children viewed in your family?
   - What are the roles of children in your family?
   - How are children cared for?
   - Who has primary child care responsibilities?
   - What happens when parents are unable to care for children?
4. What are some of the traditions, beliefs, and rituals that your family practices?
   - How do you and family members recognize/celebrate holidays, birthdays, and other occasions?
   - When did these celebrations start? By whom?
   - How have these traditions, beliefs, practices, and rituals been preserved—passed down?
5. How does your family view education and work?
   - What is your family's educational background?
   - What is your family's view of achievement?
   - What is your family's work/employment history?

6. How would you describe your family and extended family's sense of solidarity?
   - How would you describe your family's sense of "home?" Is there a central "home place?"
   - Where do your family members reside geographically?
   - How do you and your family members communicate with each other?
   - How are thoughts and feelings expressed?
   - Who can you approach in times of need?
   - What happens during times of crisis?
   - How would you describe intergenerational relationships in your family, extended family?
   - How would you describe your family and extended family's sense of solidarity?
7. What were significant transitions and/or critical life events in the history of your family, extended family?
   - What events or situations have been stressful for you and your family?
   - When these events take place how do you or family members respond?
8. How do you and family members seek help and support?
   - Where and to whom do you turn for support?
   - What social supports are available to you?
9. What is the meaning of spirituality and religion for each member of your family going back three generations?
   - How do different family members express religious and spiritual beliefs?
   - What is the level of involvement in organized religious institutions, that is, church?
   - What role does spirituality or religion play in the everyday lives of family members?
10. What are some of your family strengths?
    - What makes you feel proud?
    - How have these been passed on to you and others in your family?
    - What are your family's assets or resources?
    - What are resources or supports available in your community?

Process

The first step in constructing a CG is to introduce the genogram as a mechanism for visually exploring family history in a manner that is culturally relevant. It takes into account one's cultural values, beliefs, traditions, history, and realities. Similar to the standard genogram interview, the practitioner forms a partnership that encourages individuals or families to explore family history, recognizing that they are the experts concerning their experiences. The questions are designed to explore family history, strengths, and the broader cultural context and much of this information can be recorded within the CG. When the CG is used in conjunction with basic empathy, genuineness, and respect, it can produce good results. Table 3.1 delineates the five key areas that are explored to reveal the cultural context. Because these questions are personal, it is important to make clients feel comfortable and safe in sharing their stories and family drama. This process can take several hours depending on the size of the families. More than one interview is recommended.

Details of family structure and history over at least three generations are taken and represented in a standard format using the symbols and the basic genogram layout. Grandparents, parents, aunts, uncles, cousins, siblings, nieces and nephews, and the base household are depicted. A variety of lines are used to indicate communication patterns and the quality of relationships. Information is also gathered on significant family life cycle events such as births, deaths, marriages, divorces, cutoffs, adoptions, and separations. Other information such as family roles, extended family networks, traditions and values, solidarity, family migration, health history, education and career choices, religious affiliations and spirituality, and other life events are also recorded. This information is written in proximity to the appropriate family member or unit. For further information and instruction on how to complete a standard genogram, see McGoldrick and Gerson (1985), Stanion, Papadopoulos, and Bor (1997), and McGoldrick, Gerson, and Schellenberger (1999).

Case Example

The following section illustrates a composite family utilizing the CG. A diagram of the CG of this family can be found in Figure 3.1.

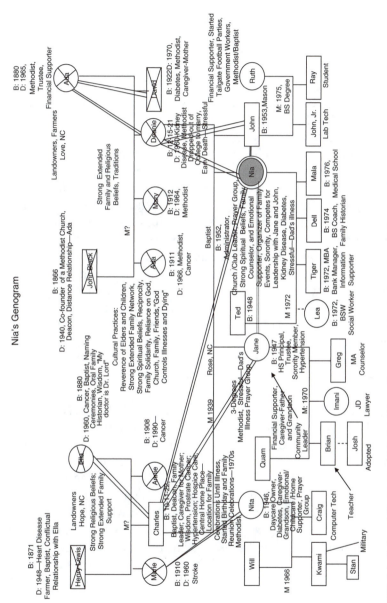

Nia's Genogram

FIGURE 3.1. Cultural Genogram Model (*Note:* B = Year of Birth; D = Year of Death; M = Year of Marriage; JD = Law Degree; NC = North Carolina; MA = Masters Degree; BSW = Bachelor of Social Work Degree)

To begin the process, the practitioner explained the purpose and procedures and provided the client Nia a list of questions. Nia reviewed the questions and indicated that she felt comfortable answering them. The practitioner and Nia explored her family and extended family composition, relationships, and cultural influences. The suggested questions and five areas were discussed and pertinent information recorded in the CG.

Nia sought help because she was feeling very sad and anxious in dealing with her father's illness and impending death. Nia is a fifty-two-year-old, well-educated, African-American, married, career-oriented woman with four adult children. She suffers from a chronic illness and over the past ten years has had to carefully attend to her personal health issues. Now her father is very ill. Nia describes herself as feeling overwhelmed and fearful, but determined to care for her eighty-year-old terminally ill father. Until his illness, Nia's father played a central role in the extended family, and his home was the base household for the family. He was the leader, provided family continuity, and organized celebrations and family events. Nia indicated that accepting the terminal condition of her father has been difficult for her and her siblings.

Nia's family had a recent crisis when they had to decide whether to place their father in a nursing home or make arrangements for him to live with one of his children. They talked about the options. One sister and a brother wanted him to be placed in a nursing home; Nia and another sister tearfully insisted upon in-home care. After much praying, crying, and emotional discussions among the siblings a family decision was made. One sister, who is also the caregiver of a grandson, agreed that their father would live with her. The family agreed to help with financial and supportive care. Through planning with their pastor and contacts in the church, an older fictive kin was hired to provide daily care for their father. On weekends Nia and her siblings share caregiving duties. During discussion, Nia realized that her family had displayed a sense of reciprocity, shared responsibility, and family duty to provide loving care for their father. The family also agreed to community services of hospice and home health care.

Nia disclosed that her father's illness had been very stressful for her family. When their father's physician asked the family to discuss with the father his terminal condition and make decisions concerning treatment and life support plans, no family member was emotionally able to do so. As a result, Nia reluctantly talked with him, and this was difficult for her. While acknowledging her pain and sadness, Nia was asked to discuss her family's belief about religion, spirituality, and death and dying. She reported that it was very difficult for the family to prepare for their father to die. The prevailing cultural and family belief is that people die when God gets ready for them. Preparing to die, in the African-American culture, means giving up and not accepting that people die in God's time. The social worker was able to highlight Nia's and her family's strong religious and spiritual belief systems and the significance of these beliefs in helping them cope with their father's terminal illness. Nia was then asked to identify the ways her spiritual beliefs and religious practices helped her cope with problems. She was encouraged to consider how she could utilize her faith and church to help her cope with this family crisis and transition. Nia stated that praying, scripture reading, and being involved in church activities strengthened her relationship with God and helped to sustain her during difficult times. She added that support from friends, sorority, club members, and extended family support networks were also helpful. The practitioner was able to help Nia identify and unleash her personal, spiritual, family, cultural strengths, and encourage her to use all the support available to her.

In constructing and reviewing Nia's genogram, it is evident that there are strong intergenerational relationships, cultural influences, and sense of family obligation and reciprocity. Though this may be viewed as a burden, Nia and her siblings feel that it is their family duty and responsibility to take care of their terminally ill father. There is a strong kinship network and a sense of commitment to giving in times of need. Strong religious values and spirituality are apparent because prayer sustains them in times of crisis. The terminal illness of the father is also causing uncertainty in family leadership and a shift in the base household. Since the terminal illness of the father, the family is uncertain about an ascribed leader. Nia continues to need support around the impending death of her father and the impact it will have on family dynamics, as well as her personal reactions.

Constructing the genogram and highlighting African-American cultural factors enabled Nia and the practitioner to discover many strengths, intergenerational family patterns, and cultural factors that can be helpful to providing services to Nia and her family. Surely the strengths identified can be instrumental in helping Nia to appreciate how she and her family have come together to cope with their father's illness. The CG also helped the practitioner to be more aware and to clearly understand all the resources that Nia has available. This is a great asset to rapport building and supportive grief and loss counseling with Nia.

Discussion and Implications for Practice

The CG, when used with African-American families, can assist in enhancing cultural understanding. It facilitates a process where both practitioners and families explore strengths, resources, and broader cultural influences. This respectful process promotes a clearer understanding and culturally competent practice. It is also empowering for clients.

This model was designed for use with African-American families but can be adapted for use with other culturally diverse families. The CG can also assist in teaching family life cycle framework in a culturally responsive manner by directing the social worker to also look at families within a cultural context. A limitation of this approach is that it does not fully explore the impact of systems outside the family. Consideration of social factors such as poverty, oppression, and social injustice, in the past and present, must also be considered. In addition, interventions, which are beyond the scope of this chapter, were not addressed. The CG, however, does lend itself to the dynamic process of engagement, assessment, and treatment. The information obtained from the CG can readily be used to help families empower themselves and help practitioners make appropriate referrals and design culturally responsive case plans.

CONCLUSIONS

The genogram is an effective assessment and therapeutic tool that focuses on intergenerational patterns and relationships among family members. When this tool is augmented to include aspects of the family's broader cultural context, it is more valuable as an instrument for culturally responsive treatment. As social workers, practitioners, and therapists make use of the CG with African-American families, culturally sensitive and appropriate practice is strengthened. It supports an understanding of family history, transactions, intergenerational relationships, cultural values, and strengths that can be utilized to encourage culturally competent assessment and treatment by professionals.

REFERENCES

Alston, R. J., & Turner, W. L. (1994). A family strengths model of adjustment to disability for African American clients. *Journal of Counseling & Development, 72(4)*, 378-383.

Bahr, K. S. (1990). Student responses to genogram and family chronology. *Family Relations, 39,* 243-249.

Barnes, S. (2001). Stressors and strengths: A theoretical and practical examination of nuclear single parent, and augmented African American families. *Families in Society, 85(5)*, 449-460.

Barth, R. (1969). *Ethnic groups and boundaries.* Boston: Little Brown.

Bean, R. A., Perry, B. J., & Bedell, T. M. (2002). Developing culturally competent marriage and family therapist: Treatment guidelines for non-African American therapist working with African American families. *Journal of Marital and Family Therapy, 28(2)*, 153-164.

Beck, R. L. (1987). The genogram as a process. *The American Journal of Family Therapy, 15,* 343-352.

Bennett, J. (1975). *The new ethnicity: Perspectives from ethnology.* St. Paul, MN: West Publishing.

Billingsley, A. (1992). *Climbing Jacob's ladder.* New York: Simon & Schuster.

Billingsley, A. (1999). *Mighty like a river: The black church and social reform.* New York: Oxford University Press.

Boyd-Franklin, N. (1989). *Black families in therapy: A multisystems approach.* New York: Doubleday.

Burton, L. (2003, May). *Homeplace in the lives of African American families.* Paper presented at the Emerging Issues in African American Family Life: Context, Adaptation, and Policy, Duke University, Durham North Carolina.

Carroll, M. (1998). Social work's conceptualization of spirituality. *Social Thought, 18(2)*, 1-13.

Congress, E. (1994). The use of culturagrams to assess and empower culturally diverse families. *Families in Society: The Journal of Contemporary Human Services, 75,* 531-540.

Cowger, C. (1994). Assessing client strengths: Clinical assessment for client empowerment. *Social Work, 39(3)*, 262-268.

DeMaria, R., Weeks, G., & Hof, L. (1999). *Focused genograms: Intergenerational assessment of individual, couples, and families.* Philadelphia, PA: Brunner/Mazel.

Dunn, A., & Dawes, S. (1999). Spiritual-focused genograms: Key to uncovering spiritual resources in African American families. *Journal of Multicultural Counseling and Development, 27*(4), 240-255.

Estrada, A., & Haney, P. (1998). Genograms in a multicultural perspective. *Journal of Family Psychotherapy, 9*(2), 55-62.

Frame, M. W. (2000). The spiritual genogram in family therapy. *Journal of Marriage and Family Therapy, 26*(2), 211-216.

Gallup, G. J., & Lindsay, D. M. (1999). *Surveying the religious landscape.* Harrisburg, PA: Morehouse Publishing.

Goldenberg, H., & Goldenberg, I. (2000). *Family therapy: An overview* (5th ed.). Pacific Groves, CA: Brooks/Cole Publishing.

Green, J. (1982). *Cultural awareness in the human services: A multi-ethnic approach.* Englewood Cliffs, NJ: Prentice Hall.

Green, J. (1999). *Cultural awareness in the human services* (3rd ed.). Boston: Allyn & Bacon.

Guerin, P. J., & Pendagast, E. G. (1976). Evaluation of family system and genogram. In P. J. Guerin (Ed.), *Family therapy.* New York: Gardner Press.

Hall, E., & King, G. (1982). Working with the strengths of black families. *Child Welfare, 61*(8), 536-544.

Hardy, K. V., & Laszloffy, T. A. (1992). Training racially sensitive family therapist: Context, content, and contract. *Families in Society, 73,* 364-370.

Hardy, K. V., & Laszloffy, T. A. (1995). The cultural genogram: Key to training culturally competent family therapist. *Journal of Marital and Family Therapy, 21,* 227-237.

Hartman, A. (1995). Diagrammatic assessment of family relationships. *Family in Society, 76*(2), 111-122.

Hartman, A., & Laird, J. (1983). *Family-centered social work practice.* New York: The Free Press.

Hill, R. (1997). *The strengths of African American families: Twenty-five years later.* Washington, DC: R & B Publishers.

Hines, P. M., & Boyd-Franklin, N. (1996). African American families. In M. McGoldrick, J. Giordano, & J. K. Peace (Eds.), *Ethnicity and family therapy* (pp. 66-84). New York: Guilford Press.

Hodge, D. R. (2001). Spiritual genograms: A generational approach to assessing spirituality. *Families in Society: The Journal of Contemporary Human Services, 82*(1), 35-48.

Keiley, M. K., Dolbin, M., Hill, J., Karuppaswamy, N., Liu, T., Natrajan, R., Poulsen, S., Robbins, N., & Robinson, P. (2002). The cultural genogram: Experiences from within a marriage and family therapy training program. *Journal of Marital and Family Therapy, 28*(2), 165-178.

Kilpatrick, A., & Holland, T. (2003). *Working with families: An integrative model by level of need* (3rd ed.). Boston: Allyn & Bacon.

Lum, D. (2000). *Social work practice and people of color: A process-stage approach* (4th ed.). Pacific Grove, CA: Brooks/Cole Publishing.

Magnuson, S., & Norem, K. (1995). Constructing genograms with lesbian clients. *Family Journal, 3*(2), 110-116.

Manns, W. (1981). Support system of significant others in black families. In H. P. McAdoo (Ed.), *Black families* (pp. 238-251). Thousand Oaks, CA: Sage Publications.

Martin, E., & Martin, J. M. (1978). *The black extended family.* Chicago: University of Chicago Press.

McAdoo, H. P. (1997). Upward mobility across generations. In H. P. McAdoo (Ed.), *Black families* (pp. 139-162). Thousand Oaks, CA: Sage Publications.

McDaniel, A. (1990). The power of culture: A review of the idea of Africa's influence on family structure in antebellum America. *Journal of Family History, 15*(1), 225-238.

McGoldrick, M. (1995). *You can go home again.* New York: Norton.

McGoldrick, M., & Gerson, R. (1985). *Genograms in family assessment.* New York: Norton.

McGoldrick, M., Gerson, R., & Shellenberger, S. (1999). *Genograms: Assessment and interventions* (2nd ed.). New York: Norton.

McGoldrick, M., Giordano, J., & Pearce, J. (Eds.) (1996). *Ethnicity and family therapy* (2nd ed.). New York: Guilford Press.

Nobles, W. (1974). Africanity: Its role in black families. *The Black Scholar, 5,* 10-17.

Nobles, W. (1991). African philosophy: Foundations of black psychology. In R. L. Jones (Ed.), *Black psychology* (3rd ed., pp. 47-63). Berkeley, CA: Cobb & Henry.

Nobles, W. (1997) African American family life. In H. P. McAdoo (Ed.), *Black families* (pp. 83-93). Thousand Oaks, CA: Sage Publications.

Pellebon, D., & Anderson, S. (1999). Understanding the life issues of spiritually based clients. *Families in Society, 80*(3), 229-238.

Pinderhughes, E. (1989). *Understanding race, ethnicity, and power: The key to efficacy in clinical practice.* New York: Free Press.

Pipes, W. H. (1997). Old time religion: Benches can't say "Amen." In H. P. McAdoo (Ed.), *Black families* (pp. 41-66). Thousand Oaks, CA: Sage Publications.

Richardson, B., & June, L. (1997). Utilizing and maximizing the resources of the African American church: Strategies and tools for counseling professionals. In C. C. Lee (Ed.), *Multicultural issues in counseling: New approaches to diversity* (2nd ed., pp. 155-170). Alexandria, VA: American Counseling Association.

Ruiz, D., & Carlton-LaNey, I. (1999). The increase in intergenerational African American families headed by grandmothers, *Journal of Sociology and Social Welfare, 26*(4), 71-86.

Schiele, J. (2000). *Human services and the Afrocentric paradigm.* Binghamton, NY: The Haworth Press.

Sowers, K. M., & Ellis, R. A. (2001). Steering currents for the future of social work. *Research on Social Work Practice, 11,* 245-253.

Stanion, P., Papadopoulus, L., & Bor, R. (1997). Genograms in counseling practice: Constructing a genogram (Part 2). *Counseling Psychology Quarterly, 10*(2), 139-148.

Sudarkasa, N. (1997). African American families and family values. In H. P. McAdoo (Ed.), *Black families* (pp. 9-40). Thousand Oaks, CA: Sage Publications.

Thomas, A. J. (1998). Understanding cultural and worldview in family systems: Use of the multicultural genograms. *Family Journal: Counseling and Therapy for Couples and Families, 6*(1), 24-32.

Waites, C., MacGowan, M. J., Pennell, J., Carlton-LaNey, I., & Weil, M. (2004). Increasing the cultural responsiveness of family group conferencing: Advancing child welfare practice. *Social Work, 49*(2), 291-300.

White, M. B., & Tyson-Rawson, K. J. (1995). Assessing the dynamics of gender in couples and families: The genogram. *Family Relations, 44,* 253-260.

Chapter 4

Health:
Intergenerational Insights and Action

Makeba Thomas
Elijah Mickel
Bernice W. Liddie-Hamilton

Children have never been good at listening to their elders, but they have never failed to imitate them.

James Baldwin

The roles of historical precedents, current culture, and family structure are significant in understanding intergenerational health. It has been suggested that African-American culture, family structure, and lifestyle, more than any other group, must be viewed in its complexity as an adaptation to conditions in the American social system (Billingsley, 1993). These conditions have often been harsh beginning with the forced removal from familiar lands and structures that supported their growth and survival to foreign shores that rendered them powerless, in a system set up to threaten every aspect of their being, offering no legal or moral protections.

This chapter begins with a review of the three historical precedents. They include the pre-Atlantic slave trade, the Middle Passage, and the Breaking-in Period. Information related to the current state of the African-American intergenerational health is explored. Next, the chapter discusses the Human Genome Project (HGP). The HGP is the most recent link requiring the Euro-scientific world to recognize the connectiveness of all human beings. Although the mapping is based upon the Western European genotype, the validity of the project's findings, in the final analysis, is the beginning of the end to phenotypical privilege. The HGP connects intergenerational health genetically to the historical precedents. Finally, African-American healing and implications for practice are also discussed. In this chapter, the authors focus on the overall health concerns of people of African descent, which began with the manner in which they were brought to the Americas and other parts of the world, identified as slaves. This includes the overall relationship between one's health status and the perceived sense of self in the social environment.

HISTORICAL PRECEDENTS

Three historical precedents impacted the current state of intergenerational health concerns among the African-American population in the United States. These precedents include the pre-Atlantic slave trade, the Middle Passage, and the Breaking-in Period. At each stage, the influence of the European culture negatively impacted the health and well-being of people of African descent. Preslavery may be defined as the period when African people were free and lived in isolated regions of Africa such that they were immune to many of the diseases in their local villages. The intrigue that led European explorers to the interior trek of Africa marked the beginning of the slave health deficit legacy (Byrd & Clayton, 2000). The tropical environment of the interior trek, where the greater part of the slave trade occurred, exacerbated the level of health threat. This tropical region, with its warmer climate, was identified as difficult to navigate and overcome with disease, most notably malaria, a parasitic disease transmitted by female mosquitoes ("Millennium Promise," n.d., www.millenium promise.org). During the roundup, captive slaves were exposed to new diseases in other regions of Africa as well as new diseases of their captors. The diseases carried by the European captors included tuberculosis, syphilis, smallpox, and measles. As a result of the roundup and treatment of captive slaves, an estimated 50 percent of those captured died before leaving Africa (Byrd & Clayton, 2000).

Those surviving the roundup faced treacherous conditions aboard slave vessels, which added to the "slave health deficit" during the

Middle Passage (Byrd & Clayton, 2000). The conditions of the Middle Passage increased the health risk and mortality rate of every captive slave aboard the vessels. Transport increased the health-related quality of life and the likelihood of death toll numbers of captive African slaves. Identified diseases during the Middle Passage included dysentery, diarrhea, ophthalmia, malaria, scurvy, worms, yaws, and typhoid fever. An excerpt from the work of Blassingame (1972) describes some of the conditions aboard the slave vessels. "The foul and poisonous air of the hold, extreme heat, men lying for hours in their own defecation, with blood and mucus covering the floor caused a great deal of sickness" (p. 7).

The conditions on the slaves' vessels not only posed a negative impact on the physical health of the slaves, but also rendered an atrocious attack on their psychological well-being. As stated by Blassingame (1972), a number of slaves were thought to develop a form of insanity owing to the inhumane conditions of the Middle Passage, while others committed suicide in an effort to resist enslavement. The conditions of the Middle Passage proved perilous to the health and lives of captured Africans.

Also important was the relationship between European physicians, referred to as slave doctors, and African slaves. The slave doctor's responsibility was to inspect slaves to ensure that they presented among the healthiest for the journey and labor that awaited them. The European view of Africans was that of nonhuman status, thus the health of Africans was merely relegated to financial gain. This relationship did not prove beneficial for the health and well-being of slaves; instead, it proved to be the beginning of a pathological viewpoint of Africans, which set a precedent for the treatment of African health upon arrival to America.

Health conditions for slaves worsened upon arrival to America. Notwithstanding the roundup and the Middle Passage, the stress of the Breaking-in Period, to include the adjustment to the new climate and exposure to new diseases, placed African health in grave danger. The stress was also related to sanitation and housing, working conditions, the dismantling of African families, brutal beatings for attempted escapes, rape, and the overall inhumane treatment in the institution of slavery. The systemic maltreatment of Africans as their land was infiltrated, to the roundup process, through the Middle Passage, and ending in enslavement in America is significant in examining the problems that currently impact the intergenerational health status of African Americans today.

The Systemic Maltreatment of Africans

The long-term systemic effect of the "slave health deficit" was articulated by Randall (2002):

> The current status of black health is based on long-term system neglect built on a "Slave Health Deficit." Another way to think about the kind of commitment needed is to consider that of the total time that a person of African descent have had a presence in the new world, 64.2% of that time was as chattel slavery and another 26.1% of that time was spent in de jure or "Jim Crow" segregation. That is, only 9.6% of the total time in the United States has persons of African descent had full legal status as citizens. From a health perspective, 64.2% of the time was spent in establishing and maintaining a health deficit and at no point has that deficit been removed. Thus the burden of a slave health deficit has been a continuous burden. (p. 4)

During their enslavement, owing to white self-interest, African Americans were subjected to hard and dirty work, much of it contributing to poor health and early death for far too many. Because they were denied entry into many health care systems and exploited by others, African Americans were bereft of health care services. Ongoing day-to-day stresses magnified the perceived crisis of illness within the African-American community. In addition, owing to the system of enslavement and its attendant vicissitudes (e.g., living in unfamiliar and hostile terrain, the breakup of the family and community structures, lack of opportunities to practice cultural values and norms, nutritional deprivation, lack of supportive services, and the harshness of being dehumanized), an ever-increasing need was created for "African Americans to utilize alternative coping mechanisms in response to their situation."

History informs us that people of African descent suffered greatly at the hands of strangers to the African culture and land. Moreover, the treatment, or nontreatment, of Africans, before, during, and upon arrival to faraway shores set a precedent for the suffering of African Americans across the United States today. The results are obvious in the continuation of disproportionate numbers of African Americans who remain adversely affected by disruption in the family structure (Staples & Johnson, 1993), denial of their former values of collective solidarity, cessation and subsequent diminution of economic opportunities, and disproportionate occurrences of diseases, including influenza, tuberculosis, pneumonia, and syphilis (Katznelson, 2005). In 2003, the death rates of African Americans were greater for diseases such as heart disease, asthma, pneumonia, cancer, cardiovascular disease, diabetes, stroke, HIV/AIDS, and homicide (African American Profile, 2003, omhrc.gov). In 2003, the infant mortality rate among African Americans was 2.4 times as high as that of the non-Hispanic population in the United States, adversely affecting the African-American unit (Centers for Disease Control, 2006). These diseases are just a modicum of the health issues that continue to significantly affect African-American families across this country, in spite of the development of highly technological advances in the area of physical and mental health.

The health issues of Africa were exacerbated during the Atlantic slave trade and its effects are evident today in the numerous health policies and practices that continue to put the African-American family disproportionately in jeopardy of failing health and consequential death. Examples of this include participation in dangerous work conditions that adversely affect their safety and expose them to health hazards, such as asbestos and other chemicals proven to cause or contribute to life-threatening illnesses. In addition, practices within the health care community often continue to offer less than adequate care for those seeking medical care, such as decisions to withhold certain treatments and exclusion of African Americans from most drug trials. Other examples include selective treatments based on the ability to pay for services (or subjective decisions in withholding treatment), a documented history of unethical practices by some physicians that have actually caused harm to those seeking assistance for the sake of medical experimentation, and bureaucratic practices that frustrate the efforts of those seeking treatment. These policies and practices are actualized in health disparities.

Intergenerational Relationships

The life of each family has its own history, character, climate, style, and its social structure. These characteristics are shaped by the larger social systems with which the family is continuing transactions. It is further shaped by its sociocultural roots and affiliations, and by the biopsychological makeup of the individuals who comprise the family system. The deprivation experienced by so many African Americans over an extended period of time has triggered many responses. One of the important reactions to this deprivation has included the reliance on intergenerational relationships. Intergenerational relationships refer to the interactions between individuals of different cohorts or generations (Troll & Bengston, 1982). When examining intergenerational relationships of African Americans, it is essential to begin with the disruption of many aspects of the lives of people of African descent.

Behavior, Genetics, and Transmissions

Just as genes are significant for intergenerational transmission of biologically based behavior, so are physical behaviors transmitted through knowledge and values. Knowledge and values are significant components of the perceptual system. These perceptions provide ways of dealing with adversity.

Historically, health and wellness belonged to the community in which there was a sense of "we-ness," there was no separating those who were ill from the community. In fact, their care and treatment was viewed as a community responsibility. Whenever African people gathered, health was a subject of discussion. It was believed that community consensus (such as prayer) worked for the health of the membership. For example, the treatment of a major illness in the community often relied on traditional health practices because no other treatment was available. See the entry in Henry McNeal Turner's "Daily Journal":

> Cure for the Whooping Cough: Take your child to some woman who is married to one of the same name and therefore did not change her name by marriage and before telling her what you

want ask her for a piece of bread and drink of water for it and give it to the child and it will cure it. (Turner, 1864)

Knowledge regarding healing is culturally based and is a continuous process handed down through the generations.

HUMAN GENOME PROJECT

The Human Genome Project (HGP) is an added tool for understanding health disparities. It can provide useful knowledge for social workers and inform their understanding of the issues involved and behavioral practices within the African-American community related to intergenerational differences, practices, and philosophy toward health and wellness. Wellness behavior from a spiritual perspective is learning about the relationship between nature and nurture. That is, learning to infuse intergenerational transmitted health with culturally transmitted behaviors.

The HGP, begun in October 1990, is a coordinated effort to describe genetic material and the concomitant sequence of the DNA in the human genome. Its major purpose is to discover and count the number of human genes and make them accessible for further study. This discovery, it is hoped, will lead to explaining the biological basis for human behavior (McInerney, 1999). Some human behaviors continue to be classified, based on race and ethnicity (e.g., health treatment disparities). It is important to understand and use the findings of the HGP because social and behavior scientists are now closer to understanding the causes for human behavior.

The ongoing work of the HGP is pertinent to social work policy and practice, with this relationship being noted in the Education Policy and Accreditation Standard (EPAS) section that describes the purposes of social work profession and social work education: "Social work education is grounded in the profession's history, purposes, and philosophy and is based on a body of knowledge, values and skills" (CSWE, 2003, p. 31). This body of knowledge is significantly impacted by the drafting of the HGP (Collins, 2001).

The search for the biological basis of intergenerational health and wellness is a significant component of the Human Genome Project. Findings of the biological basis for illness and wellness are significantly tied to this search. Just as illness is behavioral, so too is wellness. Wellness is at some point described as a resistance to disease, the ability to overcome adverse conditions. Many who support the project are looking for one gene to cure one illness and another gene as the cause for others. For those of us concerned with wellness, we see less attention paid to the search for wellness genes and health.

The intergenerational transmission of behavior is holistic and is transmitted through mind, body, and spirit. The mind and body transmission of behavior can be and will be mapped through the human genome. The documentation of the biological basis of intergenerational transmission has been codified in the outcome of the HGP. According to Dunston (2000), "Although no known biological product is encoded by much of the natural variation in the genome, it is nonetheless transmitted from generation to generation through the genome much like the genes that code for proteins, the functional products of genes." Natural variation in DNA sequences is a very rich source of information on family and population history.

Just as disease can be intergenerationally transmitted, health is also the result of intergenerational genetics. Biology (genetic) transmits the potential for some behaviors that have been identified through the human genome. According to the "Behavioral Genetics" (n.d.), "No single gene determines a particular behavior. Behaviors are complex traits involving multiple genes that are affected by a variety of other factors." A focus has been upon disease, but just as we intergenerationally transmit disease, we can also transmit the propensity for wellness.

WELLNESS AND AFRICAN-CENTERED HEALING

The experience of health and well-being is most often understood subjectively, from the perspective of the individual. The sense of wellness can be described in many different ways. Frankl (1946) describes it as having the experience of being free of disease or disability, experiencing a sense of belonging. Others have viewed wellness as having the ability to do things that are enjoyable, being creative, feeling energized and happy, being able to give and receive love, spiritual contentment, being stress free, and finding meaning in life. These perspectives of health and wellness include both the objective and subjective aspects of health and wellness, as indicated earlier. According to Gebbie, Rosenstock, and Hernandez (2003), the World Health Organizations' definition of good health is "a state of complete physical, mental and social well-being and not merely the absence of infirmity" (p. 31).The early history of health and health care in the United States focused on the physical body and its workings and did not take into account socioenvironmental and political aspects and their importance in determining wellness. Rather, health or the absence of wellness was seen as being the responsibility of the individual. For African Americans, inherent in their history was the belief in "we-ness," which was in direct contradiction to the Eurocentric notion of an "I" in relating to health and wellness. "Living in a segregated society, where racism and social inequality was evident, the relationship with the health care delivery system was virtually nonexistent and African Americans were often forced to rely on self-diagnosis and self-treatment at home" (Harper, 1990, p. 23). Anecdotal stories reflect the myriad self-treatments used by African Americans, including the use of cigar smoke to treat an earache, application of spider webs to wounds, black coffee to treat a sty, mud applied to bee stings, cooked rice, milk, and salt to "cure" diarrhea, and the use of toothpaste to avoid blisters following a burn. Again, this practice of self-reliance as a response to exclusion appears to have contributed to the various health disparities that African Americans continue to experience.

According to Mickel and Liddie-Hamilton (2002, p. 36), "The art of healing is essentially the management of the healer, the consumer and the environment." Healing mandates recognition of the intergenerational person in the environment, as well as the environment in the person. According to Mickel (1993), "It is an approach which focuses upon the relationship system, and works to modify or change those processes which detract from the strength and need fulfilling processes" (p. 36). Intergenerational healing requires a noncoercive, safe space where families can meet their basic needs. This environment is defined by families and community. The African-centered perceptual system (Mickel, 1991) provides a foundation upon which intergenerational understanding is developed. "African centered family healing presents a realistic view of the history of the family, focusing on the strengths of the family, especially noting the central role of interdependence and spirituality" (Mickel and Liddie-Hamilton, 2002, p. 36).

Ultimately, our system is designed to be need fulfilling (healthy). When the system is unhealthy (out of balance) it behaves to obtain a sense of wellness (balance). The system maintains, in its quality world, pictures of wellness. As a family, it is in our quality world that we store those memories, pictures of wellness, if you will, that can be drawn upon to provide a foundation for wellness.

When a family attempts to meet its needs, it must have the available means to meet those needs, or its behavioral system will use need fulfilling behaviors. When behaviors are constricted (unhealthy), the family will continue to behave in an attempt to perceive that it has met or is meeting its needs (quest for wellness). Our behavioral system is designed to continually move us toward wellness. This movement is influenced by our genetically driven needs. All families have the same basic needs and use the same total behavior to fulfill them. Their differences are in the genetically endowed strength of a particular need (Glasser, 1984, 1998; Mickel, 1991). Our behavior system maintains a historical record of wellness. When it is out of balance, it retrieves (sometimes with help) those instances when it was in balance and attempts to move and obtain those things that assist it to become healthy once again.

It is important that the social worker (healer) recognizes that within the process, a change in one part of the family structure causes a change in the total family (Mickel, 1990). In the final analysis, there is a dimension yet to be discussed and discovered. It is the spiritual realm. There is, in the author's opinion, an intergenerational transmission of spiritual-based total behavior. The strength of these behaviors varies (yet to be proven) from individual, family, or community to individual, family, or community.

IMPLICATIONS FOR PRACTICE

Health disparities have been defined as "gaps in the quality of health and health care across racial and ethnic groups" (Goldberg, Hayes, & Huntley, 2004, p. 4). Given the extent and effects of health disparities for African Americans, it is essential to examine a wide range of health-related factors, including social, biological, economic, and physical conditions much more closely to identify potential avenues especially appropriate for social work intervention.

A focus on health issues of the African-American family from the focal point of identifying and discussing strengths is essential in this endeavor. This should begin with an examination of the historical development of black culture, and its influence on the development of health care practices and beliefs among its members. The availability of social supports (friends, relatives, neighbors, church family), the quality and quantity of these supports, physiological risk factors, the role of sickness, alternative methodologies that do not rely solely on middle-class values, the cost of health care, the view of health and wellness that includes the total family as well as dimensions of the mind, body, and spirit are important considerations that must be incorporated into the overall assessment. This may help one avoid a pathological view of African Americans as it relates to coping mechanisms within and outside of the health care system. Additional considerations should include an interest in and understanding of the definition of community as perceived by many African Americans as well as the myriad methods employed by members of the African American to successfully navigate within their communities for services that remain, at times, unavailable, inaccessible, and unusable in the formal health care system.

Additional concerns include current social policies that threaten to adversely affect the health and health care delivery systems of members of the African-American and other poor communities. Proposed changes in Medicare and Medicaid would put pressure on states to reduce benefits, restrict eligibility, or lower payments to health care providers. Although these proposals may seem technical, they would directly and adversely affect the neediest in our society.

Cultural conflicts and differences in communication patterns continue to exist between social workers, members of the health care community, and African Americans. Methods for understanding informal and formal systems from a cultural, ethnic, and historical perspective paramount to (1) develop sensitivity for differences that exist; (2) minimize barriers to interaction; (3) strengthen health care delivery systems; and (4) further social justice for this population.

CONCLUSIONS

Genes influence health, disease, traits, and behaviors. Science is connecting the pathways that are the foundations for attributes such as handedness, cognition, diurnal rhythms, and other behavioral characteristics. Too often, research in behavioral genetics, such as that regarding sexual orientation or intelligence, has been poorly designed and its findings have been communicated in a way that oversimplifies and overstates the role of genetic factors. This has caused serious problems for those who have been stigmatized by the suggestions that alleles associated with what people perceive as "negative" physiological or behavioral traits are more frequent in certain populations. Given this history and the real potential for reoccurrence, it is particularly important to gather sufficient scientifically valid information about genetic and environmental factors to provide a sound understanding of the contributions and interactions between genes and environment in these complex phenotypes.

The role of the human genome has been to contribute sound scientific evidence to the intergenerational understanding of the role of genes and behavior to health. It reifies the end to race as a significant scientific variable. Anthropological and genotypical evidence empirically verifies the intergenerational, interconnectiveness of all human beings. Yet, genetic information has been used as a rational for discrimination. However, the HGP demands a radical restructuring of our approach to understanding human behavior and the concomitant health implications that result. This research effort, to date, has not been very inclusive of the black community. The validity of the HGP's findings is, in the final analysis, the beginning of the end to phenotypical privilege. Social workers must understand the implications of genomic information for intergenerational insights and actions.

Finally, it is important that there be robust research to investigate the implication, for both individuals and society, of uncovering any genomic contributions that there may be to traits and behaviors. The field of genomics, as well as the profession of social work, has a responsibility to consider the social implications of research into the genetic contributions to traits and behaviors, perhaps an even greater responsibility than in other areas where there is less of a history of misunderstanding and stigmatization. Decisions about research in this area are often best made with input from a diverse group of individuals and organizations.

REFERENCES

African American Profile. (2003). Health conditions: Quick facts. Retrieved November 28, 2006 from http://www.omhrc.gov/templates/browse.aspx?lvl=2& lvlID=51

Behavioral Genetics. (n.d.). Human Genome Project Information. Retrieved December 12, 2006 from http://www.ornl.gov/sci/techresources/human_Genome/ elsi/behavior.shtml

Billingsley, A. (1993). *Climbing Jacob's ladder: The enduring legacy of African American families.* New York: Simon & Schuster.

Blassingame, J. W. (1972). *The slave community: Plantation life in the antebellum south.* New York: Oxford University Press.

Byrd, W. M., & Clayton, L. A. (2000). *An American health dilemma.* Volume 1. A Medical history of African Americans and the problem of race: Beginnings to 1900. New York: Routledge Press.

Centers for Disease Control. (2006). Infant mortality statistics from the 2003 period linked birth/infant death data set. *National Vital Statistics Reports, 54*(16), Table 2.

Collins, F. S. (2001). *Remarks at the press conference announcing sequencing and analysis of the human genome.* Retrieved March 10, 2004 from http://www .genome.gov/pfv.cfm?pageid=10001379

CSWE (2003). *Handbook of accreditation standards and procedures* (5th ed.). Alexandria, VA: Author.

Dunston, G. M. (2000). The challenges and impact of human genome research for minority communities. Retrieved December 12, 2006 from http://www.ornl.gov/ sci/techresources/Human_Genome/publicat/zetaphibeta/dunston.shtml

Frankl, V. (1946). *Man's search for meaning.* Boston: Beacon Press.

Gebbie, K., Rosenstock, L., & Hernandez. L. M. (Eds.) (2003). *Who will keep the public healthy? Educating public health professionals for the 21st century.* Washington, DC: National Academies Press.

Glasser, W. (1984). *Control theory.* New York: Harper and Row.

Glasser, W. (1998). *Choice theory.* New York: HarperCollins.

Goldberg, J., Hayes, W., & Huntley, J. (2004). Understanding health disparities. *Health Policy Institute of Ohio,* November, 4.

Harper, B. C. O. (1990). Blacks and the health care system: Challenges and prospects. In S. M. L. Logan, E. M. Freeman, & R. G. McRoy (Eds.), *Social work practice with black families.* New York: Longman.

Katznelson, I. (2005). *When affirmative action was white: An untold history of racial inequality in twentieth century America.* New York: W.W. Norton Company.

McInerney, J. D. (1999). Genes and behavior. *Judicature.* Retrieved December 12, 2006 from http://www.ornl.gov/sci/techresources/human_Genome/publicat/ judicature/article4.html

Mickel, E. (1990). Family therapy utilizing control theory: A systems perspective. *Journal of Reality Therapy, 9*(1), 22-23.

Mickel, E. (1991). Integrating the African centered perspective with reality therapy/ control theory. *Journal of Reality Therapy, 11*(1), 66-71.

Mickel, E. (1993). Reality therapy based planning model. *Journal of Reality Therapy, 13*(1), 21-39.

Mickel, E., & Liddie-Hamilton, B. (2002). Family therapy in transition: African centered family healing. *International Journal of Reality Therapy, 22*(1), 34-36.

Millennium Promise. (n.d.). About malaria and how it spreads. Retrieved December 15, 2006 from http://www.milleniumpromise.org/site/PageServer?pagename= malaria_abt

Randall, V. R. (November/December 2002). Eliminating the slave health deficit: Using reparation to repair black health. *Poverty and Race, 11*(6), 3-8, 14.

Staples, R., & Johnson, L. B. (1993). Black families at the crossroads: Challenges and prospects. San Francisco, CA: Jossey-Bass Publishers.

Troll, L., & Bengston, V. (1982). Intergenerational relations throughout the life span. In J. Wolman (Ed.), *Handbook of developmental psychology.* Englewood Cliffs, NJ: Prentice Hall.

Turner, H. M. (1864). *Henry M. Turner Papers.* Box 106, Folder 1; Manuscript Division, Moorland-Spingarn Research Center, Howard University.

Chapter 5

Raising Saints in Exile: Intergenerational Knowledge Transfer in a Storefront-Sanctified Church

Deidre Helen Crumbley

The Church and its leaders were at the center of Black Philadelphia. Men, weary from work, came at night to paint the walls of
the churches. Women spent time and money buying flowers so
that the sanctuary might glorify God. And the little ones, dressed
in their best, learned ethics there on Sunday morning. On the
journey of exploring the roots of the modern Black community,
the church stands squarely by the roadside.

Ballard, 1984, p. 39

INTRODUCTION

Ballard's observation about black churches in eighteenth-century
Philadelphia also applies to the church in this study. It was founded
200 years later in the same city by a woman born just sixteen years after the Emancipation Proclamation; she would head the church until
her death at 105 years. This chapter explores the importance of this inner-city storefront-sanctified church for founding members, who arrived in the city during the Great Migration (1915-1960), and for their
offspring. It focuses on religious socialization related to personal spiritual formation, larger societal structures, and cultural traditions. Its

purpose is to identify implications for strength-based interventions that promote the resiliency of black families and communities. This chapter contains four parts: methodology, interpretive frameworks, and central concepts; the next section is an overview of the case study church; the third is a "thick" ethnographic description of its intergenerational knowledge transfer processes; and the final part ends with interventions for culturally competent social work.

HISTORICALLY EMBEDDED ETHNOGRAPHY AND THE VIEW FROM WITHIN AND WITHOUT

In this historically embedded ethnography, "thickly" documented beliefs, practices, and structures are considered against the historical backdrop of the Great Migration in which approximately 5 million rural southern blacks migrated to industrialized cities of America (Harrison, 1991, p. vii). Because of its cultural and temporal specificity, this approach does not readily produce generalizations; however, its strength lies within this limitation because its ethnographic detail and historical grounding provide a rich heuristic medium for discovering productive lines of inquiry.

Data were collected through conventional anthropological field methods of in-depth interviews, surveys, and archives. In addition, the author was raised in this church. Subsequently literature was reviewed on the implications of insider/outsider positionality (Gwaltney, 1976; Harris, 1976, 1990; Hymes, 1990; Jones, 1970; Medicine, 2001; Pike, 1997) exploring the hybridized and dialectical implications of being both within and without the ethnographic landscape (Aguillar, 1981; Bakalai, 1997; Feleppa, 1986; Halstead, 2001; Kim, 1987; Morris, Leung, Ames, & Lickel, 1999; Narayan, 1993). This study, then, employs an "observant participation" approach, requiring the researcher-member to look at the familiar with a fresh-trained eye and to assess it from the vantage of both scholar and subject (Jules-Rosette, 1975). It is neither intellectually possible nor necessarily advantageous to entirely distance oneself from a community to understand it (Spector, 1993). In addition, a responsible anthropological study of religion should access belief systems of both the researcher and the researchee (Adams, 1997).

The Sanctified Church, Religious Socialization, and Strengths-Based Assessment

"Intergenerational knowledge transference" is used interchangeably with religious socialization, that is, the internalization of divinely sanctioned values, perspectives, and behaviors grounded in beliefs about mundane and transcendent realities. Associating experience of self with "things divine, sacred and inviolable," religious communities represent landscapes of learning and support (Mattis, 2005, pp. 190, 202). Black faith communities provide unracialized contexts for self-assessment where mainstream ideals are selectively affirmed and combined with coping skills for negotiating structural racism (Boykin and Toms, 1985; Harrison-Hale, Mcloyd, & Smedley, 2004).

There is relatively little empirical data on religion and spirituality in black family life, in part, owing to European intellectual traditions that assume an antithetical relationship between material-exoteric and spiritual-esoteric ontology rather than explore their intersection (Akbar, 1985). Still, a few studies show that African Americans outscore European, Hispanic, and Asian Americans on indices of religious participation.[1] Also sparse is research on religious socialization, although Pentecostals score the highest on indices of socialization (Mattis, 2005).

"The church" shares many features of Pentecostalism but also stands in the black "sanctified church" tradition, which institutionalized selected elements of African-derived slave religion, such as spirit possession (Best, 1998; Drewal, H., 1989; Drewal, M. T., 1989; Hurston, 1981; Mbiti, 1969; Murphy, 1988; Parrinder, 1969; Ray, 2000), reinforced by holiness—Pentecostalism of the late nineteenth and early twentieth centuries (Gilkes, 1990; Hurston, 1981; Raboteau, 1978, 1993; Sanders, 1996). Sanctified churches differ from older black independent churches in organizational and worship style and offer more opportunities for female leadership (Best, 1998; Grant, 1986; Sanders, 1996; Washington, 1984). Founded in the South, sanctified churches spread North during the Great Migration, often locating in affordable rental properties, for example, storefronts (Gilkes, 1987; Harrison, 1965/1966). They were safe places of "communal parenting" where recent migrants found familiar faces, food, and ways of being while exploring their new urban setting (Sanders, 1996, p. 36).

This study employs a strengths-based approach to interventions that highlights competencies, talents, indigenous knowledge, and legacies of persistence (Maton, Schellenbach, Leadbeater, & Solarz, 2004). As strength-based assessment and constructive critique are not mutually exclusive, suggested interventions given at the end of this chapter reflect potential conflicts as well as conflations between African-American religious socialization and desired social work outcomes.

Exile and Migration As Interpretive Frameworks

> Of all the people who have come to these American shores, Black people are the only ones that never left the land of their oppression.

> Ballard, 1984

Allen E. Ballard spoke these words during a lecture at Temple University about his book *One More Day's Journey, The History of a Family and a People* (1984), a powerful blending of personal and historical narratives about the Great Migration to Philadelphia. This chapter argues that "never having left the land of their oppression" informed the rise of the case study church and continues to inform the black experience in America in the twenty-first century. Between 1940 and 1960 the South lost 3 million black Southerners who were "pulled" North by jobs created by war-related industries and stringent anti-immigration laws (Davis, 1991, p. 11; Hines, 1991, p. 218), and "pushed" out of the South by the boll weevil infestation, politicoeconomic exploitation, social marginalization, and by racial violence exemplified by the lynching of 1,663 blacks in the "Cotton South"—South Carolina, Georgia, Alabama, and Mississippi—alone between 1882 and 1930 (Tolney & Beck, 1991, pp. 22-27). In Philadelphia, the black experience of exploitation and exile assumes different institutional structures.

This notion of exile refers to a persistent awareness of being perpetually foreign, uprooted, and never at ease, and it draws on Ballard's observation that despite extensive migration blacks have never left the land of their oppression; on Sayers's analysis of African diasporan marronage in which he argues that the black experience consists of "historically recognized incidents of mass exile" (Sayers, 2006, pp. 116-117); on Sanders' exploration of "exile" among black holiness and Pentecostals as dialectical tension between "refuge and reconciliation" in which spiritual and material needs are met (Sanders, 1996, pp. ix, 36-39); and on ways saints speak of themselves as adopted Abrahamic seed (Romans 11:7), who "sojourn in a strange land" (Acts 7:6), having "no continuing city" (Hebrews 13:14).[2]

A Word About Words

Two linguistic practices in this text require clarifications. Instead of the conventional "ethnographic present," both past and present tense are used to make the point that this faith community is not static but dynamic as both religious change and continuity have occurred since its founding over fifty years ago. Second, in line with the strength-based orientation of this book, "consultant" is used in lieu of "client," the former connoting a qualified source of specialized knowledge; the latter, dependency and patronage.

CASE STUDY: THE CHURCH

Migration, the Call, and the City

Mother Brown (1879-1984) hailed from Virginia where she received a "call" that culminated in her founding the Church of Prayer Seventh Day (COPSD).[3] It grew from a handful to about one hundred adults and children consisting of five major extended families. Undaunted by the pronouncement of Baptist church leaders that "God never called a woman to preach," this separated mother of two answered her call, settling in Philadelphia in 1914, the year World War I began, where, by 1930, over two-thirds of the black population had been born in Virginia, North and South Carolina, and Georgia, some were recruited to work in steel mills and other industries (Ballard, 1984, pp. 8, 185).

However, they had not left the land of their oppression. The Southern economy they left behind had been built on chattel slavery; the wealth of Philadelphia had been built on slave-produced rum and provisioning slave ships (Ballard, 1984). Fleeing Southern racial terrorism, they arrived in a city with a history of whites burning down black orphanages and churches (Ballard, 1864). Southern sharecropping and domestic work salaries of $2.50 per week[4] had their Philadelphia analogue in the concentration of black labor in blue collar and service industries, exacerbated by a steady flow of industry from the black city core to less accessible white suburbs (Ballard, 1984; Hershberg, Burnstein, Ericksen, Greenberg, & Yancey, 1979). As late as 1910, the state of South Carolina had only one public black high school (Ballard, 1984); however, blacks migrating to Philadelphia encountered de facto segregated schools that formed the foundation for today's tiered racialized educational system (Ballard, 1984).

Health discrepancies were also met by Great Migration blacks in Philadelphia, where infant mortality was twice as high for blacks as whites. The death rate from tuberculosis, four times higher, was not unconnected to a population density averaging 28.2 whites per acre, but 111 per acre for blacks (Ballard, 1984). Founding saints recall that the National Guard was called out in 1944 to protect black trolley car drivers recently hired by the city of Philadelphia.[5] Police brutality was so normative that this author recalls Mother Brown cautioning the saints to discipline their children because if they didn't beat their children "the police would" and would use "rubber hoses" instead of the plastic belts that parents regularly used.

Initially, Philadelphia may have been perceived as an oasis of greater possibilities and less rampant racial violence, but, while saints had left the South, they had not left the United States. As the black-other in America (Pandian, 1985), they had to negotiate racialized hierarchies both north and south of the Mason Dixon Line. Nevertheless, the beliefs, values, and practices of the church would provide useful tools for negotiating new Northern racial practices and socioeconomic hierarchies.

Religious Beliefs and Practices

Key religious beliefs and practices of the church include being saved, divine law, embodiment of the spirit, biblical authority, divine revelation, adept veneration, and testifying. "Being saved" entails being "in but not of" the world (St. John 17:11, 16), and, in the words of Mother Brown, "wearing the world as a loose garment." When founding saints were not at home, work, school, or school-related events they were at church where three services were held during Sabbath, sunset

Friday to sunset Saturday, on Sunday afternoons, and Tuesday eve-nings. "Keeping the law" means complying with select Levitical laws, the Decalogue, and teaching of Jesus. Keeping the law yields bless-ings (Deuteronomy 28:1-14) and forms a covenant with God through adoption into the lineage of Abraham (Romans 11:17-24). Excellence in achievement, at work and school, is another consequence of keep-ing the law. Although some evangelical traditions reject education as an impediment to salvation, in the church it is the means to, and a sign of, being "the head and not the tail" (Deuteronomy 28:13).

Being Holy Ghost–filled is expressed behaviorally through a "changed life" because "faith without works is dead" (James 2:20) and mystically through embodied power to heal, speak in tongues, and "shout" the holy dance. The divine is also known through the ulti-mate authority of biblical revelation. Biblical literalism is selective; not all Levitical laws are observed and New Testament passages that taught women to be "silent" in church and "submissive" to husbands (1 Timothy 2:11-15; Ephesians 5:22) are offset by Galatians 3:28, as-serting that in Christ there is "neither male nor female."

As scripture is "of no private interpretation" (2 Peter 1:20), revela-tion is ongoing and "cumulative" rather than fixed or "perfect." Saints work out their "own salvation with fear and trembling" (Philippians 2:12); yet, some saints possess higher status owing to spiritual gifts. Mother Brown, the ultimate arbiter of doctrine was revered for her anointment, gift of "preaching the word," and "getting a prayer through." All saints regardless of status are free to testify, which opens formu-laically with, "Giving honor to God, the pastor, deacons, and saints" and concludes with, "Pray for me that I will grow stronger in the Lord." In the intervening narrative, saints recount personal experiences and share life's tragedies, challenges, problems, achievements, and aspirations.

Organizing Principles: Seniority, Gender, and Kinship

Gender, age, and kinship are intertwined themes in church organi-zation. For the founding generation, ritual and political power were centralized in a female founder ritually assisted by "head saints" from each major extended family. Duties of their husbands, the "deacons," were money related; males were only minimally involved in the ritual realm. Biblical references to Lois, Eunice (2 Timothy 1:5) and Priscilla (Act 18:26; Romans 16:3; 2 Timothy 4:19; 1 Corinthians 16:19), and Judge Deborah (Judges 5:7) along with the living role model of Mother Brown countered scripturally based female subordination (1 Timothy 2:11-15; Ephesians 5:22).

The importance of age as an organizing principle is demonstrated by Mother Brown remaining head of the church until her death at 105 years. After her demise, founding generation saints, both male and female, assumed the spiritual leadership of the church as its "elders." In the church, "family" and "church" conflate literally, since the church has grown along family lines, and symbolically, since members are addressed with kinship terms, for example, "Brother James" and "Mother Brown." Youths are responsive to the parental gaze of both fictive and biological kin, and deferring to age is normative; adults are answered, "Yes ma'am or sir," never simply, "Yes."

As in all families, interactions are lived out within the confluence of compassion, cooperation, and conflict. During the founding generation, conflict took the form of ongoing interfamily comparisons and quest for favor with the pastor; compassion and cooperation were demonstrated by saints helping each other with housing, transportation, employment, and care for the sick. In addition, the church treasury has continued to be a source of interest-free loans.

INTERGENERATIONAL KNOWLEDGE TRANSFERENCE

The church was a space apart where youths were protected from dangers and distractions of the city and were socialized to be saints. North Philadelphia, where the church was located and most founding saints resided in the 1940s and 1950s, had meager community resources and a high unemployment rate. Youths could readily get caught up in street life and by being in the wrong place at the wrong time could become victims of police brutality. All adult saints are parented, not with biological relations alone. Family, culture, and God were conflated into a unitary experience of a reality in which boundaries were clearly set and divinely sanctioned. Learning this distinctive view of reality entailed intergenerational knowledge transfer in matters pertaining to spiritual formation, social structures, and cultural legacy.

Spirituality

For founding saints, spiritual formation, the shaping of one's relationship to the divine and the mundane transformed children into "saints." Youths learned the significance of divine law, comportment of "holiness," embodying Spirit, biblical reflection, and "testifying." Early on, children learned to note the exact time the sun set on Friday, Sabbath evening, to defer to elders, and to read food labels lest they eat "unclean meat," fostering attention to detail, codes of respect for self and others, and care of the body.

Founding saints also instructed youths in the importance of "holiness" in all aspects of life in the way one dressed, talked, and socialized (Titus 2:3). These practices kept children away from potentially dangerous settings and fostered the habit of considered decision making even when unfashionable. Spiritual formation also entailed learning that God was imminent, accessible, and it "filled" the saints with mystical power expressed through shouting and glossolalia, "speaking in tongues." Children attended the same services as adults, so they grew up watching, internalizing, and eventually replicating their singing, shouting, speaking in tongues, and praying in the spirit.

Youths participated in "devotional services," played instruments in "the band," and were affirmed for memorizing lengthy Bible passages and inspirational "pieces." As soon as a child would repeat words, he or she repeated, "Jesus wept" (John 11:35), in front of a supportive congregation. Youths learned how to reflect on scripture during Bible study, which encouraged public-speaking skills based on intellectual discipline. As they grew up hearing their parents "testify" in time their own formulaic testimonies expanded into personal narratives of divine intervention.

Social Reality

Founding saints transferred to the next generation knowledge of, and strategies for negotiating, racialized structures in American society. White people and white racism were never the explicit subject of sermons; however, vicissitudes of "living while black" in America shaped the content of our prayers and made our ideology of excellence quite functional. When children of the church returned from school recounting cases of everyday racism on the part of both teachers and students, first generation saints reminded them that as Holy Ghost–filled, commandment keeping "saints of the Most High God," they were the "head and not the tail" and "above" those who belittle them.

Founding saints imparted poignant critiques and proactive responses to social inequity. Distinguishing between socially ascribed status and true human worth, youths learned to respectfully address a man who was a janitor during the week and as "deacon" on Sabbath. Similarly, notions of black intellectual inferiority were countered by the notion of academic excellence as a sign of salvation and commandment keeping. For founding generations, youths were expected to earn only As and Bs; earning a C grade was tantamount to failure. This valuing of education helped church youths accrue invaluable cultural capital; although they were not allowed to join the scouts or attend movies, they could visit museums, theaters, and other "educational" sites. It also dovetailed well with educational opportunities fostered by the 1954 Supreme Court anti-segregation ruling. In line with the Great Migration pattern of black labor being concentrated in blue collar and unskilled labor, most male saints worked in factories and female saints "did days work" cleaning houses; however, they instilled in their offspring the determination to "do better."

As television and newspapers were not forbidden, youths were aware of the events unfolding around them: the shadow of Hiroshima and associated regular "duck and cover" air raid drills;[6] McCarthy's anti-communist witch hunt; the Korean War (1950-1953) and the Vietnam War (1954-1975); and the lynching and mutilation of fourteen-year-old Emmett Till in Money, Mississippi (1955). Youths were taught to endure and consider these events within, and subordinate them to, larger contexts of sacred history.

Cultural Legacy

Although the larger Philadelphia social structure was white-dominated, urban, and racialized, the church was a working model of black self-determination and institutional autonomy, flavored with African-American southern rural themes. Here, youths received proper "home training" in self-comportment, linguistic proprieties, and deference to age. Youths internalized a culture of "church food" highlighting the best of black southern cuisine (Dodson and Gilkes, 1995, pp. 519-536). At the church, they also learned their cultural history as the curriculum of newly integrated public schools in the 1950s and 1960s did not reflect cultural legacies of its diversifying student population.

The author recalls instruction from a songbook that included "Old Black Joe" and Stephen Foster's "Old Folks at Home," including the line, "Oh darkies, how my heart grows weary." Historical icons were white, including females such as Betsy Ross and Florence Nightingale, with the exception of Marian Anderson, a Philadelphia native, and Paul Robeson, until his political activism and the McCarthy witch hunts led to the loss of his passport, career, and health. The rare reference to blacks in history was an uncritical allusion to slavery that ascribed more shame to the enslaved than the enslaver.

In contrast, Mother Brown, born just sixteen years after the Emancipation Proclamation, related the stories her mother told her about bush arbor prayer meetings where enslaved black people turned up a pot to "catch the noise" so that slaver owners would not hear and beat them for it the next day.

Mother Brown, usually emotionally self-contained, shed tears once when relating a narrative of black mothers wailing as their children were sold away from them on the auction block. Thus, slavery was no sign of shame to black people, but it said a lot about the humanity of those who blithely destroyed black families for personal gain that their children would inherit. Such explicit allusions to racial injustice from the pulpit were extremely rare, but because founding saints and their children spent most of their leisure time together with one another, oral traditions of life "down home" were regularly passed down.

Founding generations modeled gender practices that were at variance with those of white male dominated structures in the larger American society. From deference shown, the female pastor-founder, first generation youths learned that women can be leaders; from male and female elders who now provide church leadership, today's youths learn that men and women can share leadership. Although validated by scripture (Galatians 3:28), the practice of black men and women sharing authority in the church is also rooted in west African dual-sex legacies, reinforced by the equalizing impact of structural racism on African-Americans gender practices (Gilkes, 1994).

DISCUSSION: IMPLICATIONS
AND INTERVENTIONS

Implications: Negotiating Persistent Exile

Strengths-based assessment and structural critique are not mutually exclusive. The church has its strengths and its weaknesses. It has functioned as a cultural critique of, and alternative to, an experience of exile, wherein a "world of sin" and the world of racialized social structures are conflated. Ideologically affirming and culturally safe, the church is where there are no penalties for being black and poor and where saints wade in the same streams of African-American cultural history and societal experience. Saints also share a clearly defined and divinely sanctioned worldview shaped by the religious legacy of the sanctified church.

However, like all refugees, the church runs the risk of further insulating the already marginalized. Without the ballast of alternative perspectives and disinterested critique, a community of exile can become an alienated group disassociated from the rest of humanity. For this reason, some second generation saints children "left the church" as adults working hard to learn the social skills for interacting with people in the world. Indeed, becoming an anthropologist was one way the author came to understand the church as a particular expression of a universal human quest for meaning and power.

Despite obvious limitation of self-marginalization, this little storefront church of a hundred souls has produced public school teachers, administrative level civil servants, nurses, social workers, computer/hi-tech specialists, a nationally recognized radio programmer, a college administrator, and two PhDs. As recently as 2002, every college age student in the church had matriculated.[7] Still, saints respect different educational capacities of the youths as indicated by an enthusiastic round of applause given to a young brother with learning disabilities when he testified that he had completed his associates degree at Philadelphia Community College. Second-generation saints have also established an "education fund" for college students, and individual saints continue the informal practice of "putting a few dollars in the hand" of students when they reach benchmarks of academic achievement.

Still, given the historical specificity of this study, what can a social worker take from this case study to enhance cultural competence when working with African-American families in the twenty-first century? Over fifty years have passed since the founding of the church, but as Ballard noted, black people still have not left the land of their oppression. African Americans negotiate social structures in which race and poverty are so intimately woven that the predominance of blacks devastated by the 2005 Hurricane Katrina has reinvigorated the concept of caste as a heuristic category for investigating the status and inequality in twenty-first century America (Harrison-Hale et al., 2004).

The twenty-first century is marked by exacerbated educational, health, and socioeconomic discrepancies. Shockingly, in the wealthiest nation in the world, 59 percent of all Americans will live at least one year below the official poverty line, but, nine of every ten black Americans will know poverty during their working adult years. Federal housing, tax, transportation, zoning, and mortgage lending policies[8] have contributed to increased black school segregation from 62 percent in 1968 to 70 percent by 1999. Over half of black families fell below the asset poverty level in 1999, more than twice the number of white families. White-inherited *wealth* is three times greater than blacks, and the racial wealth gap between blacks and whites who were twenty to twenty-nine years old in 1984 had increased by $23,926 by 1994 (Shapiro, 2004).

Health discrepancy statistics at the start of the twenty-first century indicate that when compared to whites, blacks, for whom the unemployment rate in 2002 was twice that of whites, are twice as likely to die from diabetes; have twice the infant mortality rate; black pregnant women are twice as likely to start prenatal care in the third trimester or not at all, and black women, though 20 percent less likely to be diagnosed with breast cancer, are 30 percent more likely to die from it.[9] Also, black patients with early stage lung cancer are less likely than whites to undergo life-saving surgery and subsequently are more likely than whites to die of the disease. This had been related, not to differences in socioeconomic status, insurance, general health, or access to medical care, but to doctors not recommending surgery to blacks as often as to whites (Grady, 1999).

This last example suggests that not only have material structures of exile persisted since the church was founded, but they continue to be undermined by personal attitudes and acts of everyday racism. Thus, the intentional intergenerational transfer of knowledge about spiritual formations of self, negotiating racialized social hierarchies, and community-sustaining cultural legacies are as important today as it was a half century ago—if not more so. Black faith communities, then, continue to be reservoirs of divinely sanctioned and culturally valued resources for culturally competent intervention.

Interventions: Critical and Strengths-Based

The goal of the questions that follow is to help social work professionals carefully and critically explore the religious community of their consultant for ways religious beliefs and practices might inform social work outcomes:

1. What are the specific formal and informal religious behaviors and affiliations of your consultant? Two caveats: A person who appears "unchurched" may pray privately and/or rely heavily on the prayers of a relative. In addition, multiple affiliations and religious traditions may coexist.
2. What do you know about his or her particular faith tradition? *The Black Church in the African American Experience* (Lincoln & Mamiya, 1990) consists of useful denominational profiles. The documentary *Let the Church Say Amen* (Petersen, 2005) highlights the impact of small urban storefront churches, such as the case study discussed earlier, on black urban dwellers. *African American Islam* (McCloud, 1995) is another accessible informational resource.[10]
3. What is your consultant's relationship to the leaders of the faith community and how might these authority figures including unofficial "church mothers" become allies in developing effective interventions?
4. How does the religious community function as a sociocultural unit, how does your consultant function within its structures, and how might this promote his or her accruing of cultural capital and social skills?
5. To what degree does this faith community represent physical and emotional safe space for your consultant and how might you build on this?

6. How do the beliefs and practices of the faith inform your consultant's construction of self in relation to the larger society? For example, in contrast to the church, is formal education denigrated, and, if so, what are implications for educational goal setting? If women play important leadership roles, how can you draw on this to enhance the self-esteem of a female consultant? If, like the church, his or her faith community represents both a culturally affirming and world-rejecting community, what additional social skills might your consultant need to function in the larger world? How might millenarian anticipation impact long-term goal setting?

7. Finally, what is your own religious enculturation and how might it affect your perception of the faith community as an asset or a deficit in intergenerational knowledge transfer? Is religion an "opiate of the masses" for you? Might expressive elements of black worship be off-putting to someone from your religious background? Can you temporarily bracket your religious worldview and immerse yourself in the religious worldview of your consultant as a participant-observer?

Today, the church, although less world rejecting, is still small, millenarian, and is still raising black saints in exile. Other black communities of faith are doing the same, passing on spiritual values, social knowledge, and cultural legacies for negotiating racialized hierarchies. Resourceful professionals who are willing to learn about and draw upon such cultural reservoirs will enhance their strategies for effective and competent intervention with black families for whom faith is a core value.

NOTES

1. National statistics from a 1999 survey indicate that 89 percent of African-American self-identify as religious, and African-American adolescents, compared to their European, Hispanic, and Asian-American peers are disproportionately likely to pray and report the importance of religion in their lives (Mattis, 2005, p. 191).

2. All biblical citations are from the King James Version.

3. All names are pseudonyms to protect the privacy of the saints.

4. Personal interview. Elder Bernice Nicholson Crumbley, June 20, 2006.

5. Personal interview. Elder Bernice Nicholson Crumbley, June 20, 2006; Elder Ruth Nicholson Hector, March 6, 2006. Also see Ballard, 1984, pp. 75-79, 83-85.

6. 1951 official Civil Defense Administration film featuring Bert, the safety conscious turtle. Accessed July 13, 2006 from http://www.archive.org/details/ Duckand C1951

7. Personal interview. Bernice Crumbley, May 20, 2002.

8. According to a well-regarded Federal Reserve Board study, blacks are denied home loans 80 percent more often than equally qualified whites, although both met the same creditworthiness test (Shapiro, 2004, pp. 109-110).

9. Office of Minority Health: African American Profiles. Accessed July 24, 2006 from http://www.omhrc.gov/templates/browse.aspx?lvl=2&lvlID=51

10. Your knowledge of consultants' religious culture will not only command their respect but also promote rapport.

REFERENCES

Adams, W. R. (1997). Introduction. In F. Salamone & W. R. Adams (Eds.), *Explorations in Anthropology and Theology* (pp. 1-22). Lanham, MD: University Press of America.

Aguilar, J. L. (1981). Insider research: Ethnography of a debate. In *Anthropologists at home in North America* (pp. 15-26). Cambridge: Cambridge University Press.

Akbar, N. (1985). Our destiny: Authors of a scientific revolution. In H. P. McAdoo & J. L. McAdoo (Eds.), *Black children: Social, educational, and parental environments* (pp. 18-31). Beverly Hills, CA: Sage Publications.

Bakalaki, A. (1997). Students, natives, colleagues: Encounters in academia and in the field. *Cultural Anthropology, 12*(4), 502-526.

Ballard, A. B. (1984). *One more day's journey: The story of a family and a people.* New York: McGraw-Hill.

Best, F. O. (1998) Breaking the gender barrier: African-American women and leadership in black holiness-Pentecostal churches 1890-Present. In F. O. Best (Ed.), *Black religious leadership from the slave community to the million man march: Flames of fire* (pp. 153-168). Lewiston, NY: Edwin Mellen Press.

Boykin, A. W., & Toms, F. D. (1985). Black child socialization: A conceptual framework. In H. P. McAdoo & J. L. McAdoo (Eds.), *Black children: Social, educational and parental environments* (pp. 33-51). Beverly Hills, CA: Sage Publications.

Davis, D. (1991). Toward a socio-historical and demographic portrait of twentieth-century African Americans. In A. Harrison (Ed.), *Black exodus. The great migration from the American South.* Jackson, MS: University Press of Mississippi.

Dodson, J. E., & Gilkes, C. T. (1995). There's nothing like church food: Food and the U.S. Afro-Christian tradition: Re-membering community and feeding the embodied S/spirit(s). *Journal of the American Academy of Religion, 63*(3), 519-536.

Drewal, H. (1989). Art or accident: Yoruba body artist's and their deity Ogun. In S. T. Barnes (Ed.), *Africa's Ogun: Old world and new* (pp. 235-260). Bloomington, IN: Indiana University Press.

Drewal, M. T. (1989). Dancing for Ogun in Yorubaland and in Brazil. In S. T. Barnes (Ed.), *Africa's Ogun: Old world and new* (pp. 199-234). Bloomington, IN: Indiana University Press.

Feleppa, R. (1986). Emics, etics, and social objectivity. *Current Anthropology, 27*(3), June, 243-255.

Gilkes, C. T. (1987). Some mother's son and some father's daughter: Gender and biblical language in Afro-Christian worship tradition. In M. R. Miles, C. W. Atkinson, & C. H. Buchanan (Eds.), *Shaping new vision: Gender and values in American culture* (pp. 73-95). Ann Arbor, MI: UMI Research Press.

Gilkes, C. T. (1990). Together and in harness: Women's tradition in the sanctified church. In M. R. Malson, E. Mudimbe-Boyi, J. F. O'Barr, & M. Wyer (Eds.), *Black women in America: Social science perspectives* (pp. 223-244). Chicago: University of Chicago Press.

Gilkes, C. T. (1994). The politics of silence: Dual-sex political systems and women's traditions of conflict in African-American religion. In P. E. Johnson (Ed.), *African-American Christianity* (pp. 80-109). Berkeley, CA: University of California Press.

Grady, D. (1999). Racial discrepancy is reported in surgery for lung cancer. Accessed July 24, 2006 from http://query.nytimes.com/gst/fullpage.html?sec=health&res=9A04E6D61230F937A257C1A96F958260

Grant, J. (1986). Black women and the church. In J. B. Cole (Ed.), *All American women: Lines that divide, ties that bind* (pp. 359-369). New York: Free Press.

Gwaltney, J. L. (1976). On going home again—Some reflections of a native anthropologist. *Phylon (1960), 37*(3), 236-242.

Halstead, N. (2001). Ethnographic encounters: Positionings within and outside the insider frame. *Social Anthropology, 9*(3), 307-321.

Harris, M. (1976). History and significance of the emic/etic distinction. *Annual Review of Anthropology, 5,* 329-350.

Harris, M. (1990). Emics and etics revisited. In *Emics and etics: The insider outsider debate* (pp. 48-61). Newbury Park, CA: Sage Publications.

Harrison, A. (1991). *Black exodus. The Great Migration from the American South.* Jackson, MS: University Press of Mississippi.

Harrison, I. (1965/1966). Storefront religion as a revitalization movement. *Review of Religious Research, 7,* 160-165.

Harrison-Hale, A. O., Mcloyd, V. C., & Smedley, B. (2004). Racial and ethnic status: Risk and protective processes among African American families. In K. I. Maton, C. J. Schellenbach, B. J. Leadbeater, & A. L. Solarz (Eds.), *Investing in children, youth, families and communities: Strengths-based research and policy.* Washington: American Psychological Association.

Hershberg, T., Burnstein, A., Ericksen, E. P., Greenberg, S., & Yancey, W. L. (1979). Tale of three cities: Blacks and immigrants in Philadelphia: 1850-80, 1930, and 1970. *Annals of the American Academy of Political and Social Science, 44*(1), 55-81.

Hines, D. C. (1991). Black migration to the urban midwest. In J. W. Trotter (Ed.), *The Great Migration in historical perspective: New dimensions of race, class, and gender.* Bloomington, IN: Indiana University Press.

Hurston, Z. N. (1981). *The sanctified church.* Berkeley, CA: Turtle Island.

Hymes, D. H. (1990). Emics, etics, and openness: An ecumenical approach. In T. N. Headlandm, K. L. Pike, & M. Harris (Eds.), *Emics and etics: The insider outsider debate* (pp. 120-125). Newbury Park, CA: Sage Publications.

Jones, D. (1970). Toward a native anthropology. *Human Organization, 29*(4), 251-259.

Jules-Rosette, B. (1975). *African apostles: Ritual and conversion in the church of John Maranke.* Ithaca, NY: Cornell University Press.

Kim, C. S. (1987). Can an anthropologist go home again? *American Anthropologist, 89*(4), 943-946.

Lincoln, C. E., & Mamiya, L. H. (1990). *The black church in the African American experience.* Durham, NC: Duke University Press.

Maton, K., I., Schellenbach, C. J., Leadbeater, B. J., & Solarz, A. L. (2004). Strengths-based research and policy: An introduction. In K. I. Maton, C. J. Schellenbach, B. J. Leadbeater, & A. L. Solarz (Eds.), *Investing in children, youth, families and communities: Strengths-based research and policy.* Washington: American Psychological Association.

Mattis, J. S. (2005). Religion in African American life. In V. C. McLoyd, N. E. Hill, & K. A. Dodge (Eds.), *African American family life: Ecological and cultural diversity.* New York: Guilford Press.

Mbiti, J. S. (1969). *African religions and philosophy.* London: Heinemann.

McCloud, A. B. (1995). *African American Islam.* New York: Routledge.

Medicine, B. (2001). Ella C. Deloria: The emic voice. In S-E. Jacobs (Ed.), *Learning to be an anthropologist and remaining "native"* (pp. 269-287). Urbana, IL: University of Illinois Press.

Morris, M. W., Leung, K., Ames, D., & Lickel, B. (1999). Views from inside and outside: Integrating emic and etic insights about culture and justice judgment. *Academy of Management Review, 24*(4), 781-796.

Murphy, J. M. (1988). *Santeria: An African religion in America.* Boston: Beacon Press.

Narayan, K. (1993). How native is a "native" anthropologist? *American Anthropologist, 95*(3), 671-686.

Pandian, J. (1985). *Anthropology and the Western tradition: Toward an authentic anthropology.* Prospect Heights, IL: Waveland Press.

Parrinder, G. (1969). *West African religion.* London: Epworth Press.

Petersen, D. (2005). *Let the church say amen:* The Film Movement Series. Year 3. Available online at: www.filmmovement.com

Pike, K. L. (1997). On the emics and etics of Pike and Harris. In *Emics and etics: The insider outsider debate* (pp. 28-47). Newbury Park, CA: Sage Publications.

Raboteau, A. J. (1978). *Slave religion: The invisible institution in the antebellum south.* New York: Oxford University Press.

Raboteau, A. J. (1993). Introduction. In C. Johnson (Ed.), *God struck me dead: Voices of ex slaves.* Cleveland, OH: Pilgrim Press.

Ray, B. C. (2000). *African religions: Symbol, ritual, and community.* Upper Saddle River, NJ: Prentice Hall.

Sanders, C. (1996). *Saints in exile: The holiness-Pentecostal experience in African American religion and culture.* Oxford: Oxford University Press.

Sayers, D. O. (2006). Diasporan exiles in the Great Dismal Swamp, 1630-1860. *Transforming Anthropology, 14*(1) April, 10-20.

Shapiro, T. M. (2004). *The hidden cost of being African American.* New York: Oxford University Press.

Spector, J. D. (1993). *What this awl means: Feminist archaeology at a Wahpeton Dakota village.* St. Paul, MN: Minnesota Historical Society Press.

Tolnay, S., & Beck E. M. (1991). Rethinking the role of racial violence in the Great Migration. In A. Harrison (Ed.), *Black exodus* (pp. 20-35). Jackson, MI: University Press of Mississippi.

Washington, J. R. (1984). *Black sects and cults.* Garden City, NY: University Press of America.

Chapter 6

The Increase in Intergenerational African-American Families Headed by Grandmothers

Dorothy S. Ruiz*
Iris B. Carlton-LaNey

This chapter analyzes census data on grandparent heads of house-hold. Information on African-American grandparents, grandmothers in particular, is the focus of this analysis. The data include a profile of African-American grandparent householders, reasons for the increase in households headed by grandparents, challenges and problems, living arrangements/household characteristics, and implications for practice. African-American children are more likely to live in the home of their grandparents than are white or Hispanic children. In 1993, 12 percent of African-American children lived in the home of their grandparent in comparison to 4 percent for whites and 6 percent for Hispanics. The increased complexity of intergenerational households, along with a variety of social problems, suggests that new strategies must be developed to help these families cope.

Demographic and socioeconomic trends have drastically influenced the structure of African-American families (Billingsley, 1992). Along with structural family changes, there has been a concomitant change in

*Dorothy S. Ruiz is on leave from the University of North Carolina at Charlotte. This work was supported by the National Institutes of Health, National Institute on Aging, Behavior and Physiology in Aging Grant No. 2T32AG00029. *Journal of Sociology and Social Welfare,* December, 1999, Volume XXVI, Number 4. Reprinted with permission.

Social Work Practice with African-American Families

grandmothers' roles and responsibilities (Burton & Dilworth-Anderson, 1991; Dilworth-Anderson, 1992). Historically, grandparents, especially grandmothers, have played very instrumental roles in African-American extended families. Frazier (1939, 1966) appropriately described African-American grandmothers as *guardian of the generations*. They have served as guardians and caretakers for their own children, grand-children, and great-grandchildren as well as for their parents and a host of other extended and fictive kin. The grandmother represents wisdom and strength while serving as the keeper of family values such as respect, religion, love, and community. The grandmother re-minded family members of their obligations, virtues, and goals. As we approach the new millennium and a new census cycle, it seems timely that we examine the primacy of the African-American grand-mothers' roles as healers, stabilizers, nurturers, and hopegivers.

In spite of the changing demographics and contemporary role re-sponsibilities of African grandmothers raising grandchildren, there has been little empirical research on this topic. Although it is generally understood that the grandmother role has roots in the African culture, there is very little emphasis on these issues in the literature on slavery, reconstruction, and Jim Crowism. Perhaps, this is because the grand-mother role was such an integral part of the structure, function, and survival of African-American families. It would be difficult to over-look the current stressors and problems that grandparents, especially grandmothers, experience while functioning as surrogate parents to their grandchildren. A number of reasons account for the prevalence of grandmothers in this role. With the increase in AIDS, crime, crack-cocaine usage, and incarceration of adult children, custodial grand-mothers face escalating financial and social burdens as we enter the twenty-first century. There is an urgent need for social scientists to study aggressively the scope, nature, and magnitude of the issues in-volved. In an effort to ensure strong and healthy families, we need to understand how these and other social and public health problems influ-ence the daily lives and well-being of African-American grandparents.

RESEARCH PERSPECTIVES

Although little is known about the contemporary roles of African-American grandmothers, grandparenthood, in general, has been explored from a number of different perspectives. Studies of white grandparents have a tendency to focus on describing different types of grandparents and examining the meaning of the grandparent role (McCready, 1985; Neugarten & Weinstein, 1964); whereas studies of African-American grandparents focus on grandparents acting in the role of parent (Burton, 1992; Burton, Dilworth-Anderson, & Merriwether-deVries, 1995; Flaherty, Tacteau, & Garver, 1987; Minkler & Roe, 1993; Pearson, Hunter, Cook, Ialonga, & Kellam, 1997; Pearson, Hunter, Ensminger, & Kellam, 1990). Some studies on African-American grandparents have emphasized the importance of family structure and grandparenting (Burton, 1995; Burton & Dilworth-Anderson, 1991; Wilson, 1984).

AFRICAN-AMERICAN GRANDPARENTS AS SURROGATE PARENTS

Studies have documented grandparents, especially grandmothers, acting as surrogate parents in the case of divorce or desertion (Ahrons & Bowmen, 1982; Cherlin & Furstenberg, 1968; Gladstone, 1988; Johnson, 1985), drug addiction (Burton, 1992; Minkler, 1991; Minkler, Rose, & Price, 1992), and adolescent pregnancy (Burton, 1992, 1995; Burton & Bengtson, 1985; Flaherty, Facteau, & Garver, 1987; Furstenberg, 1980; Ladner & Gourdine, 1984; Thomas, 1990). A recurrent theme in the literature suggests that grandparents have a positive impact on the lives of their grandchildren. The study by Solomon and Marx (1995) found that children raised solely by their grandparents did well in relation to children in families with one biological parent present. Generally, grandparents in the role of parents seem to have a positive influence on the lives of their grandchildren.

Grandparents who have sole parental responsibilities for taking care of their grandchildren experience a number of psychological and social problems. Shore and Hayslip (1990a, 1990b) found that grandparents who had assumed total responsibility for caring for their grandchildren had reduced scores on three out of four measures of psychological well-being, including satisfaction with the grandparent role, perceptions of grandparent-grandchild relationships, and overall well-being. Burton (1992) found that caring for grandchildren produced considerable stress for grandparents. She also noted that grandparents reported feeling depressed or anxious most of the time. However, in spite of the anxiety, researchers have found that surrogate parenting role for grandparents to be both challenging and rewarding (Burton & deVries, 1993).

Challenges Faced by African-American Grandmothers

Multigenerational households are not a new phenomenon in African-American families. Although the present trend is seen in all racial and ethnic groups, the increase in grandmother-headed households is most prevalent among inner-city, low-income African-American families. A number of reasons have contributed to the increase in grandparents assuming the role of parent. As stated earlier, social problems such as AIDS, divorce, teenage pregnancy, abandonment, imprisonment, and abuse have contributed to family disruption, leaving dependent children without reliable adult supervision and guardians. These problems, exacerbated by a lack of support from formal and informal support systems, make this group particularly vulnerable.

Despite the social, economic, and health problems grandmothers face, they accept the parental responsibility of taking care of a vast number of children who would otherwise become wards of the state or "victims of the streets." Suddenly forced to sacrifice both time and money in order to care for their grandchildren, many grandmothers maintain one or more full- and/or part-time jobs. Some are forced to return to work after retirement. Often, African-American grandmothers are responsible for taking care of several generations, including nieces and nephews, as well as parents and other elder family members.

Households Maintained by African-American Grandparents

According to the U.S. Bureau of the Census (1994), African-American children are more likely to live in the home of their grandparents than are white or Hispanic children. In 1993, 12 percent of African-American children lived in the home of their grandparent(s), in comparison to 4 percent for whites and 6 percent for Hispanics. Similar proportions of African-American, white, and Hispanic grandchildren had only their mother present. African-American grandchildren were more likely than other grandchildren to have a parent present at all and less likely to have both parents living with them in the grandparents' home. In 1993, 53 percent of the 1.3 million grandchildren had only their mother present, 39 percent had neither parent present, 4 percent had both parents, and 4 percent had only their father present. White and Hispanic children were equally as likely to have both parents present as to have neither present (U.S. Bureau of the Census, 1994).

The U.S. Bureau of the Census (1994) further reports that there were 2.1 million families maintained by grandparents with grandchildren present. More than one-half of the grandparents' homes were maintained by both the grandmother and the grandfather, 43 percent by only the grandmother, and 4 percent by only the grandfather. The families maintained by white grandparents were more likely to have both grandparents present (63 percent) than were families maintained by African-American grandparents (35 percent). In African-American families, only the grandmother was more likely to head the family (62 percent as compared with 33 percent for white families). Households headed by African-American grandparents increased from 30 percent in 1991 to 43 percent in 1994. Among families of Hispanic origin, 53 percent were maintained by both parents and 43 percent by the grandmother only (Table 6.1).

AFRICAN-AMERICAN FAMILIES AND CHILDREN

Living Arrangement of Children

The proportions of families with children have declined for both the African-American and white populations. In 1970, nearly 2 million African-American families were childless; by 1993, this number had increased nearly 75 percent to 3 million. The comparable increase for whites was 47 percent from approximately 21 million to nearly 31 million families. In 1993, non-Hispanic white families were less likely than African-American families to include children. The living arrangements of children are directly related to the marital patterns of the adult population. In today's society, children are less likely to live in traditional two-parent families and are much more likely to reside in single-parent families. This reflects the increase in divorce as well

TABLE 6.1. Grandchildren of the Householder, by Presence of Parents, Race, and Hispanic Origin: 1994, 1990, 1980, and 1970 (numbers in thousands)

Living Arrangement	1994				1990	1980	1970
	Total	White	Black	Hispanic[a]	1990	1980	1970
Children under 18	65,508	54,795	11,177	9,496	62,276	63,369	69,276
Grandchildren of householder	3,735	2,122	1,451	539	3,155	2,306	2,214
Percentage of children under 18	5.4	3.9	13.0	5.7	4.9	3.6	3.2
Children with both parents present	460	336	69	101	467	310	363
Children with mother only present	1,764	971	733	237	1,563	922	817
Children with father only present	175	142	23	43	191	86	76
Neither parent present	1,359	673	627	158	935	988	957
Percent	100.0	100.0	100.0	100.0	100.0	100.0	100.0
With both parents present	11.7	15.8	4.8	18.7	14.8	13.4	16.4
With mother only present	47.2	45.8	50.5	44.0	49.5	40.0	36.9
With father only present	4.7	6.7	1.6	8.0	6.1	3.7	3.5
With neither parent present	36.4	31.7	43.2	29.3	29.6	42.8	43.2

Source: For 1970 and 1980 data: U.S. Bureau of the Census, 1970 Census of Population, PC(2)-4B, Persons by Family Characteristics. 1980 Census of Population, PC80-4B. For 1994 data: U.S. Bureau of the Census, 1990 Census of Population, Current Population Reports, Population Characteristics, P20-484, Marital Status and Living Arrangements: March 1994.

[a]Persons of Hispanic origin may be of any race.

as the number of never-married women who have children. Since 1970, the proportion of children living with two parents has declined for both African Americans and whites. In 1993, approximately 10 million African-American children or 94 percent lived with at least one parent. Of those living with at least one parent, 58 percent lived with their mother only and 38 percent lived with both parents. In contrast, 16 percent of non-Hispanic white children lived with their mother only and 80 percent lived in two-parent families. A similar proportion of both African-American and non-Hispanic white children (approximately 3 percent) resided with their father only (U.S. Bureau of Census, 1994).

The proportion of all children living with one parent more than doubled from 12 percent in 1970 to 27 percent in 1993. The proportion of children living with mother only almost doubled for African Americans, from 29 percent in 1970 to 54 percent in 1993, and more than doubled for whites, from 8 to 17 percent in 1993. African-American children were almost three times more likely than non-Hispanic white children to have an absent parent, 64 and 21 percent, respectively (Table 6.2).

TABLE 6.2. Living Arrangements of Children Under 18 Years by Race and Hispanic Origin: 1991, 1980, and 1970 (Numbers in thousands. Excludes persons under 18 years old who were maintaining households or family groups and spouses)

Living Arrangement	1991	1980	1970	Percentage Distribution		
				1991	1980	1970
All Races						
Children under 18 years	65,093	63,427	69,162	100.0	100.0	100.0
Living with						
Two parents	46,650	48,624	58,939	71.7	71.7	85.2
One parent	16,624	12,466	8,199	25.5	19.7	11.9
Mother only	14,608	11,406	7,452	22.4	18.0	10.8
Father only	2,016	1,060	748	3.1	1.7	1.1
Other relatives	1,428	1,949	1,547	2.2	3.1	2.2
Nonrelatives only	383	388	477	0.6	0.6	0.7
White						
Children under 18 years	51,918	52,242	58,790	100.0	100.0	100.0
Living with						
Two parents	40,733	43,200	52,624	78.5	82.7	89.5
One parent	10,142	7,901	5,109	19.5	15.1	8.7
Mother only	8,585	7,059	4,581	16.5	13.5	7.8
Father only	1,557	842	528	3.0	1.6	0.9
Other relatives	787	887	696	1.5	1.7	1.2
Nonrelatives only						

TABLE 6.2 *(continued)*

Living Arrangement	1991	1980	1970	Percentage Distribution		
				1991	1980	1970
Black						
Children under 18 years	10,209	9,375	9,422	100.0	100.0	100.0
Living with						
Two parents	3,669	3,956	5,508	35.9	42.2	58.8
One parent	5,874	4,297	2,996	57.5	45.8	31.8
Mother only	5,516	4,117	2,783	54.0	43.9	29.0
Father only	358	180	213	3.5	1.9	2.3
Other relatives	565	999	820	5.5	10.7	8.7
Hispanic Origin[a]						
Children under 18 years	7,462	5,459	4,006[b]	100.0	100.0	100.0
Living with						
Two parents	4,944	4,116	3,111	66.3	75.4	77.7
One parent	2,222	1,152	(NA)	29.8	21.1	(NA)
Mother only	1,983	1,069	(NA)	26.6	19.6	(NA)
Father only	239	83	(NA)	3.2	1.5	(NA)
Other relatives	230	183	(NA)	3.1	3.4	(NA)
Nonrelatives only	66	8	(NA)	0.9	0.2	(NA)

Source: For Hispanic data for 1970: U.S. Bureau of the Census, 1970 Census of Population, PC(2)-IC, Persons of Spanish Origin. For 1993 data: U.S. Bureau of the Census, 1990 Census of the Population, Current Population Reports, Population characteristics, P20-484, Marital Status and Living Arrangements: March 1994.

Note: NA = Not available.

[a]Persons of Hispanic origin may be of any race.

[b]All persons under 18 years.

Children's living arrangements differed based on age groups. Children under six years were less likely than older children to live with both parents. Approximately one-third of African-American children under six lived in two-parent families, in comparison to 37 percent of six- to eleven-year-old, and 39 percent of twelve- to seventeen-year-old African

Americans. In contrast, 80 percent of non-Hispanic white children in two age groups under age six and six to eleven years old, and 77 percent of twelve to seventeen years old lived in two-parent families in 1993. Fifty-eight percent African-American children living with their mother only, in 1993, resided with never-married mother. This was more than three times the percentage of non-Hispanic white children (17 percent). Both African-American and non-Hispanic white (35 percent) children under six who lived with their mother only were more likely than older children to live with a never-married mother (U.S. Bureau of the Census, 1994).

CHILDREN LIVING IN GRANDPARENT HOUSEHOLDS

Since 1970, the proportion of children living with their grandparents has increased from 3 to 12 percent for African Americans and from 1 to 4 percent for whites. A larger proportion of non-Hispanic white (22 percent) than of African-American children under age six (4 percent) living in grandparent households lived with both parents in these households. In 1993, a similar proportion of African-American children (53 percent) and of non-Hispanic white children (46 percent) who lived in grandparent households also lived with their mother only. Nearly 40 percent of African-American children compared with 26 percent of non-Hispanic white children living with the grandparent did not have either parent present in the household. Approximately two-thirds of African-American children under six who lived in their grandparents' homes lived with their mother only. This was one and a half times the proportion of six- to eleven-year-olds (45 percent) and almost twice the proportion of twelve- to seventeen-year-olds, 38 percent (U.S. Bureau of the Census, 1994).

Profile of African-American Grandparent Householders

In 1993, the median age of the African-American grandparent householder was about fifty-five years. Approximately one-half of all African-American grandchildren lived in a household where the grandparent householder had at least a high school education, and some 7 percent where the grandparent householder had at least a bachelor's degree. Grandparent households tended to be concentrated inside central cities of metropolitan areas (62 percent). About one-fourth lived in the suburbs of metropolitan areas (23 percent) and some 20 percent lived in nonmetropolitan areas. In 1991, some 20 percent of all African-American children under age five with working mothers were cared for by their grandparents. Many working mothers are turning to grandparents for help. In the same year, a similar proportion of African-American (12 percent) and white (8 percent) preschoolers whose mothers worked were cared for by their grandparents in their grandparents' home (U.S. Bureau of the Census, 1991).

IMPLICATIONS FOR PRACTICE

The sociodemographic information presented in this chapter is useful to construct profiles of grandmothers that can be matched with various interventions. Furthermore, demographic and mortality changes in African-American families have led to greater diversity in the structure and age composition of intergenerational families (Hunter, 1997). The increased complexity of intergenerational households, along with a variety of social problems, suggests that new strategies need to be presented to help these families cope. Societal ideals of the traditional grandmother role must be altered to reflect a more realistic image. The resulting image includes an intensification of both expectation and obligation. Many of the grandmothers who have total responsibility for taking care of their grandchildren did not anticipate this role as part of their life's course, and have mixed feelings about fulfilling these obligations. Their new role is met with myriad emotions that run the gamut from anger and resentment to relief and peaceful resolvement. As one grandmother, participating in a Head Start program in a major East Coast city, succinctly described it, "You do what you have to do" (Bell & Smith, 1996, p. 18).

Incorporating an Afrocentric perspective, which identifies and builds on family strength, is fundamental to the strategies that social workers and other human service professionals must use to assist African-American grandmothers and intergenerational or "skipped generation" families. Hill (1997) noted that the culture of resilience that characterizes African-American families comes largely from the African tradition. Furthermore, he indicated, role flexibility or the interchangeability of parental roles and functions among adult family members especially grandmothers has been critical to the survival of the African-American family (Hill, 1977; Wilson, 1991). Danzy and Jackson (1997) note that the African-American perspective of child care by family members other than the biological parents is "family preservation," not "child placement." Grandmothers are especially valued in the African-American family. Their many roles include providing financial and emotional support, and helping to maintain continuity while functioning as the anchor and reservoir of advice and resources. As the primary caregiver for grandchildren whose parents are not available, the custodial grandmother needs support, encouragement, and reassurance in her role. The following discussion looks at services for intergenerational households headed by African-American grandmothers as they take on the parenting role for their children's children. Three target groups of direct or indirect intervention—grandmothers, children, and organizations/institutions—are identified. Organizations such as county Departments of Social Services, Departments of Aging, schools, churches, fraternities and sororities, as well as boys' and girls' organizations are included in this category. Many of the resilient programs presented can be useful for any intergenerational family or household.

Direct strategies or interventions provide ways to immediately influence the lives of these individuals while the indirect strategies are supportive and involve coordinating and linking caregivers and groups together. Pinson-Millburn, Fabian, Schlossberg, and Pyle (1996) indicate that these interventions require the least amount of professional intervention time, but are effective outreach methods. Furthermore, they provide needed supportive tangible and intangible resources while giving reassurance to the grandmothers that their responsibilities and needs are being considered and respected.

Hill (1997) identifies both direct and indirect resilient programs across the country that provide successful intervention and services for grandmothers and their grandchildren. While many of these programs were not designed specifically to serve grandmothers and their custodial grandchildren, they nonetheless, can help to meet many of the needs that these families have. These resilient programs are based on an Afrocentric paradigm that emphasizes a collective conceptualization of human beings and their group survival. Essentially, the sense of the collectivity must be axiomatic to the design of resilient programs that target this population. These resilient programs inform, encourage, and support grandmothers and their grandchildren alike.

Resilient programs that directly target the children while indirectly serving the grandmothers are most beneficial. Project 2000 (in the Baltimore/Washington area) is an example of a resilient program that is designed to provide early intervention to enhance the academic performance of African-American boys, especially those from families headed by women. Project 2000 provides adult male volunteer teacher assistants in grades one through three. These men assist with classroom instruction while serving as role models (Hill, 1997) to young boys. Jawanza Kunjufu has also designed a program that targets African-American male youth. The program called SIMBA is a comprehensive male socialization program developed to prepare boys, ages from seven to nineteen, for the rites of passage to responsible manhood and fatherhood. Similarly, Leonard Long, through the West Dallas Community Centers (WDCC) Rites of Passage Project, seeks to help males and females ages from nine to twelve who are at risk of early parenting, drug abuse and criminal activity. The WDCC Rites of Passage Project, incorporated in 1988, uses an Afrocentric and holistic approach in building self-esteem, self-image enhancement, leadership development, and cultural inculcation (Long, 1992). The Senior Parents' Group is an example of a resilient program that targets the grandmothers and indirectly serves the children. Established by the Chicago Child Care Society, the Senior Parents' Group was established for parents, grandparents, and other relatives who were having child rearing difficulties in middle-age or later life. The goals of the group include helping members to master the common developmental tasks of their age and assisting them in coping with the stresses of being primary child rearers at their age in life (Stokes & Greenstone, 1981).

Burton (1992) found that grandparents frequently requested respite care for parenting. Out of guilt that they may have failed once as parents and out of fear that child protective services may remove the children from their care, these grandparents are often reluctant to seek opportunities for a break. Furthermore, Burton indicated that grandparents requested information on parenting and child-rearing strategies. Any resilient program designed to meet these needs should be holistic and should build on the natural helping system that is in the community. This would eliminate the need to utililize the formal system and would decrease the grandmothers' fear of being judged by the service provider.

The African-American family tradition may mitigate against seeking help outside the nuclear family and extended family network. A history of abuse from formal professional helpers and the residuals of segregation require that social workers and other professional helpers look for ways to involve natural helpers in meeting these families needs (Taylor, Chatters, & Jackson, 1993). This history may also suggest the need for vigorous outreach through familiar and trusted institutions and organizations. In some cases, women's groups including secret orders such as the Eastern Star or the Daughters of Zion may be the source of that informal support. McPhatter (1997) notes that workers must include neighborhoods and communities as vital aspects of their practice domain. They must be intimately familiar with valuable resources offered by churches and other resilient community-based programs. Where no organizations or programs exist, social workers and other service providers must facilitate their creation. Establishing organizations of community helpers is part of the African tradition of mutual aid and support. The process of creating self-help is empowering. Moreover, it is likely to produce a program that is more effective than those that are adaptations of programs designed for the majority culture and replicated for African Americans.

In conclusion, it is anticipated that this chapter will refocus our attention and shed some light on one of our most valued, yet neglected and vulnerable populations—African-American grandmothers. Their intervention constitutes a protective factor that serves everyone in society, particularly the African-American community. It is, therefore, critical that we continue to examine strategies for serving these women and their grandchildren.

REFERENCES

Ahrons, C. R., & Bowman, M. E. (1982). Changes in family relationships following divorce of adult child: Grandmothers's perceptions. *Journal of Divorce, 5,* 49-64.

Bell, M., & Smith, B. (1996). Grandparents as primary caregivers. *The Council for Exceptional Children,* 18-19.

Billingsley, A. (1992). *Climbing Jacob's ladder: The enduring legacy* of *African American families.* New York: Simon & Schuster.

Burton, L. M. (1992). Black grandparents rearing children of drug-addicted parents: Stressors, outcomes, and social service needs. *The Gerontologist, 32,* 744-751.

Burton, L. M. (1995). Intergenerational patterns of providing care in African-American families with teenage childbearers: Emergent patterns in an ethnographic study. In V. L. Bengtson, K. W. Schaie, & L. M. Burton (Eds.), *Adult intergenerational relations: Effects of societal change* (pp. 79-96). New York: Springer Publishing Company.

Burton, L. M. & Bengtson, V. L. (1985). Black grandmothers: Issues on timing and continuity of roles. In V. L. Bengtson & J. F. Robertson (Eds.), *Grandparenthood.* Beverly Hills, CA: Sage Publications.

Burton, L. M., & deVries, C. (1993). Challenges and rewards: African American grandparents as surrogate parents. In L. Burton (Ed.), *Families and aging.* Amityville, NY: Baywood Publishing Company.

Burton, L. M., & Dilworth-Anderson, P. (1991). The intergenerational roles of aged black Americans. *Marriage and Family Review, 16,* 311-330.

Burton, L. M., Dilworth-Anderson, P., & Merriwether-deVries, C. (1995). Context and surrogate parenting among contemporary grandparents. *Marriage and Family Review, 20*(3/4), 349-366.

Cherlin, A., & Furstenberg, F. F. (1986). Grandparents and family crisis. *Generations, 10*(4), 26-28.

Danzy, J., & Jackson, S. (1997). Family preservation and support services: A missed opportunity for kinship care. *Child Welfare, 76,* 31-44.

Dilworth-Anderson, P. (1992). Extended kin networks in black families. *Generations, 16*(Summer), 29-32.

Flaherty, S., Facteau, L., & Garver, P. (1987). Grandmother functions in multi-generational families: An exploratory study of black adolescent mothers and their infants. *Maternal Child Nursing Journal, 16,* 61-73.

Frazier, E. F. (1939). *The Negro family in the United States.* Chicago: University of Chicago Press.

Frazier, E. F. (1966). *The Negro family in the United States.* Chicago: University of Chicago Press.

Furstenberg, F. F. (1980). Burdens and benefits: The impact of early childbearing on the family. *Journal of Social Issues, 36,* 64-87.

Gladstone, J. W. (1988). Perceived changes in grandmother-grandchild relation following a child's separation or divorce. *The Gerontologist, 28,* 66-72.

Hill, R. (1997). *The strengths of African American families: Twenty-five years later.* Washington, DC: R&B Publishers.

Hunter, A. (1997). Counting on grandmothers: Black mothers' and fathers' reliance on grandmothers for parenting support. *Journal of Family Issues, 18,* 251-269.

Johnson, C. L. (1985). Grandparenting options in divorcing families: An anthropological perspective. In V. L. Bengtson & J. F. Robertson (Eds.), *Grandparenthood* (pp. 81-96). Beverly Hills, CA: Sage Publications.

Ladner, J., & Gourdine, R. (1984). Intergenerational teenage motherhood: Some preliminary findings. *A Scholarly Journal of Black Women, 1*(2), 22-24.

Long, L. (1992). An Afrocentric intervention strategy. In L. Goddard (Ed.), *An African-centered model of prevention for African-American youth at high risk* (pp. 87-92). Rockville, MD: U.S. Department of Health and Human Services. Center for Substance Abuse Prevention Technical Report-6.

McCready, W. C. (1985). Styles of grandparenting among white ethnics. In V. L. Bengtson & J. F. Robertson (Eds.), *Grandparenthood.* Beverly Hills, CA: Sage Publications.

McPhatter, A. (1997). Cultural competence in child welfare: What is it? How do we achieve? What happens without it? *Child Welfare, 76,* 255-278.

Minkler, M. (1991). *Health and social consequences of grandparent caregiving.* Paper presented at Gerontological Society of America, San Francisco.

Minkler, M. (1993). *Grandmothers as caregivers: Raising children of the crack cocaine epidemic.* Newbury Park, CA: Sage Publications.

Minkler, M., Rose, K., & Price, M. (1992). The physical and emotional health of grandmothers raising grandchildren in the crack cocaine epidemic. *The Gerontologist, 32,* 752-760.

Neugarten, B. L., & Weinstein, K. (1964). The changing American grandparents. *Journal of Marriage and the Family, 26,* 199-204.

Pearson, J. L., Hunter, A. G., Cook, J. M., Ialonga, N. S., & Kellam, S. G. (1997). Grandmothers involvement in child caregiving in an urban community. *The Gerontologist, 37,* 650-657.

Pearson, J. L., Hunter, A. G., Ensminger, M. E., & Kellam, S. G. (1990). Black grandmothers in multigenerational households: Diversity in family structure and parenting involvement in the Woodlawn community. *Child Development, 61,* 434-442.

Pinson-Millburn, N., Fabian, E., Schlossberg, N., & Pyle, M. (1966). Grandparents raising grandchildren. *Journal of Counseling and Development, 74,* 584-554.

Shore, R. J., & Hayslip, J. B. (1990a). *Comparisons of custodial and noncustodial grandparents.* Paper presented at Gerontological Society of America, Boston.

Shore, R. J., & Hayslip, J. B. (1990b). *Predictors of well-being in custodial and non-custodial grandparents.* Paper presented at American Psychology Association, Boston.

Solomon, J. C., & Marx, J. (1995). To grandmother's house we go: Health and school adjustment of children raised solely by grandparents. *The Gerontologist, 35*(3), 386-394.

Stokes, J., & Greenstone, J. (1981). Helping black grandparents and older parents cope with child rearing: A group method. *Child Welfare, 60,* 691-701.

Taylor, R., Chatters, L., & Jackson, J. (1993). A profile of familial relations among three-generation black families. *Family Relations, 42,* 332-341.

Thomas, J. (1990). The grandparent role: A double bind. *International Journal of Aging and Human Development, 31,* 169-171.

Wilson, M. (1984). Mothers and grandmothers perceptions of parental behavior in three-generational black families. *Child Development, 55,* 1333-1339.

Wilson, M. (1991). The context of the African American family. In J. Everett, S. Chipungu, & B. Leashore (Eds.), *Child welfare and Afrocentric perspective.* New Brunswick, NJ: Rutgers University Press.

U.S. Bureau of the Census. (1991). Census of the Population, Current Population Reports, Population Characteristics, P20-461, Martial Status and Living Arrangements: March 1991.

U.S. Bureau of the Census. (1994). Census of Population, Current Population Reports, Population Characteristics, P20-484, Marital Status and Living Arrangements: March 1994.

Chapter 7

Intergenerational Family Influences on the Education of African-American Children

Sheara A. Williams
Monica Terrell Leach
Laurie B. Welch

Education is the single most consistent and powerful instrument for the advancement of an individual and a people.

Johnnetta B. Cole

INTRODUCTION

Educational attainment is highly valued in the United States and considered by many to be the surest pathway to self-sufficiency and social equality. The education of African-American children as a group has been characterized by a complex history of social inequality, racism, discrimination, and yet progress. It has only been 110 years (*Plessey v. Ferguson,* 1896) since African Americans received the legal right to receive an education in this country and fifty-two years since being allowed to "learn" with Americans of other races (*Brown v. Board of Education, Topeka,* 1954). Given this history, the attainment of education has been both a challenge and a highly valued dream for African-American families that transcends across generations (for a review, see Leach & Williams, in press).

The African-American family has been able to sustain itself through a strong kinship bond, typified by extended family members from

Social Work Practice with African-American Families

multiple generations. Grandparents, particularly, "have often raised their grandchildren as a result of African tradition, family survival during slavery, and the parents' search for economic opportunity" (Hunter & Taylor, 1998 cited in Goodman & Silverstein, 2002, p. 677). Therefore, the intergenerational practice of African-American grandparents raising their grandchildren is not a new phenomenon—it has a long-standing history.

That said, grandparent caregivers are faced with a number of challenges when raising school-aged grandchildren—one of the most difficult being the inability to provide tangible educational support to promote their academic success (Strozier, McGrew, Krisman, & Smith, 2005). In the twenty-first century, this kinship arrangement is necessitated, and further complicated, by a plethora of social issues including the incarceration of parents, child abuse and family violence, HIV/AIDS, substance abuse, single-adolescent parenting, and high divorce rates (Barnes, 2001; Ruiz & Carlton-LaNey, 1999). Social issues such as these have been identified in the literature as risk factors for school failure (Richman, Bowen, & Woolley, 2004), grade retention (Berrick & Barth, 1991; Eckenrode, Laird, & Doris, 1993), and behavioral problems (Lansford et al., 2002). The prevalence of this intergenerational family structure and its historical practice in the African-American community, coupled with the challenges grandparents face when parenting grandchildren, have important implications for the school experiences, academic achievement, and educational attainment of African-American children.

The purpose of this chapter is to examine the influences of the intergenerational family structure on the education of African-American children. We begin with a presentation of key terms and issues related to the topic, followed by a presentation of statistics, trends, and a summary of relevant research. Next, we highlight select programs specifically designed to assist intergenerational families in meeting their broad range of challenges, particularly related to the education of their children, and conclude the chapter with implications for school social work practice.

KEY TERMS AND RELEVANT ISSUES

Grandparent *caregiving*—also known as intergenerational caregiving or *reparenting*—has been defined in several ways in research. Although there is no clear consensus regarding the actual title, researchers agree that grandparent caregiving generally involves grandparents serving as the primary kinship care provider for their grandchildren, usually following a disruptive event (e.g., parental incarceration, drug addiction, or death) that hinders the parenting abilities of the biological parents (Fuller-Thomson & Minkler, 2000; Heywood, 1999; Pruchno, 1999; Waldrop & Weber, 2001). This designation includes those grandparents who have legal custody of their grandchildren as well as those who do not (Heywood, 1999). The following terms are frequently used to define grandparents as care providers:

1. Custodial grandparents
2. Surrogate grandparents
3. Grandparent caregivers
4. Secondary caregivers
5. Coresident grandparents

Within the intergenerational family structure, boundaries are blurred as grandparents assume heavy parental roles at more than one point in the life cycle. For this reason, grandparent caregiving is also said to be *time disordered* or *off-time* parenting in that grandparents are caring for a younger generation during a time where other individuals at similar points in life are not (Aldous, 1995; Carter & McGoldrick, 2005; Smith & Dannison, 2003). Minkler (1999) specifically identified grandmothers as *women in the middle* in that these women often simultaneously care for their own children and grandchildren and often have to combine work outside the home with parenting obligations.

This unique intergenerational family structure is often defined in accordance with those individuals involved in the child's life. Specifically, it involves the extent to which the biological parents are involved in the child's life (Brown, 2003; Fuller-Thomson, Minkler, & Driver, 1997; Heywood, 1999; Minkler, 1999). The two terms that are most frequently used to define this family structure are

1. *Skipped generation households:* Households in which the biological parent is not present in the home and kinship care is provided only by the grandparent (e.g., custodial grandparent).
2. *Three-generational family system:* Both grandparent and parent provide support and caregiving for a child (e.g., coresident grandparent).

Given the number of individuals involved in a multigenerational family system, various integral relationships form surrounding the care of the primary child. In their exploration of intergenerational family dynamics, Weber and Waldrop (2000) specifically identified four ongoing and significant relationships that are typical in multigenerational families, with the following two types specific to grandparent caregivers:

1. *Grandparent-grandchild relationship:* The relationship of the grandparent(s) assuming a primary caregiver role to the grandchild. This relationship is often formed as a result of traumatic events and is based on care and security.
2. *Parent-adult child relationship:* The relationship of the grandparent and his or her own child (the parent of the grandchild in care). This relationship is often characterized by power struggles, usually involving child custody arrangements and manipulation of resources.

These relationships, and the level of involvement of specific family members, will vary from family to family; however, the child remains the central figure through which these relationships are formed and maintained. With regard to grandparent involvement, the extent of the relationship can range from limited contact to that of primary caregiver. In addition, the level of involvement often depends on circumstances surrounding the parenting abilities of the biological parent. In reviewing the literature surrounding intergenerational caregiving, Reynolds, Wright, and Beale (2003) identified three main types of grandparent involvement:

1. *Involuntary caretaking:* Grandparents become the primary caregiver of their grandchild and often assume this role with little or no forewarning (e.g., death of the biological parent, teenage pregnancy).
2. *Voluntary caretaking:* Grandparents choose to assume the primary caregiver role to their grandchild owing to the inability of the biological parent to fulfill the role. Often the grandparent feels more available to assist in such situations, for instance, when grandparents have retired.

3. *Participatory caretaking:* Grandparents who voluntarily or involuntarily participate in the caregiving of the grandchild. Grandparents' involvement may range from being highly involved to extremely limited.

Grandparents who become primary caregivers for their grandchildren often face stressors that go beyond those typically faced by most biological parents. These stressors stem from within and outside of the family structure and have implications for caregiving. For example, grandparent caregivers may feel a sense of burden in their role of primary caregiver. In their research examining support structures for grandparent caregivers, Strozier and colleagues (2005) specifically identified three ways in which this burden was experienced and perceived: (1) *objective burden* is the perceived disruption of the physical or material aspects of a caregiver's life; (2) *subjective demand burden* is the extent to which the caregiver perceives the caregiving responsibilities to be overly demanding; and (3) *subjective stress burden* is the perceived emotional impact of caregiving responsibilities. In addition, Pruchno (1999) examined the experiences of Caucasian and African-American grandparent caregiving and identified three main stressors that frequently impact custodial grandparenting: (1) *contextual stressors,* which are dangers associated with the surrounding environment (e.g., neighborhood crime); (2) *familial stressors,* which include the stress associated with having to provide for multiple kin and the subsequent drain on the family income—this can be exacerbated by the adult child's behavior (e.g., addiction or incarceration); and (3) *individual stressors,* which depict the stress associated with a loss of personal time and the struggle to balance work and family life.

As previously mentioned, many grandparent caregivers do not anticipate becoming a parent a second time around. Despite this, formal and informal mechanisms currently exist that take grandparents into consideration first when biological parents cannot fulfill their obligations. The Kinship Care Act of 1997 was amended to Title IV of the Social Security Act and placed grandparents first in line as potential foster and adoptive parents for grandchildren who, for safety reasons, have been removed from the biological parents' care (U.S. Senate, 1997). Aldous (1995) identified feelings of obligation as a norm within multigenerational relationships. Despite their desire or ability to help in raising their grandchildren, grandparents often feel a sense of duty in assisting close relatives when they are in need. With the growing number of grandparent caregivers, practitioners should be aware of such mechanisms that may impact the lives of their clients. Practitioners should also be familiar with the unique structure and relationship dynamics of multigenerational families in order to build positive working relationships and increase chances of success.

STATISTICS, TRENDS, AND RESEARCH SUMMARY

Statistics and Trends

According to the 2000 U.S. Census, approximately 5.8 million grandparents reside with grandchildren who are under age eighteen (Simmons & Dye, 2003)—a substantial increase from the 4.6 million *coresident* grandparents in 1997, as reported by Bryson and Casper (1999). Among *all* coresident grandparents in the year 2000, 42 percent (or 2.4 million) were the primary caregivers for their grandchildren in which 52 percent of African-American grandparents were the primary caregivers for their grandchildren (Simmons & Dye, 2003). In fact, African-American grandparents are four times more likely to reside with grandchildren than their non-Hispanic white counterparts (Saluter, 1996). To the African-American family, this is not a new practice; such families have a long history of providing intergenerational kinship care owing to family crises and family preservation.

These trends have significant socioeconomic implications for the African-American family. Turner (1995) observed most grandparent-headed households to occur in urban/inner-city settings, while Simmons and Dye (2003) found the highest percentage of grandparent caregivers living below the poverty line and in the southern region of the United States. On the basis of data extracted from a nationally representative survey, Minkler and Fuller-Thomson (2005) examined conditions among more than 42,500 African-American grandparents aged forty-five years and older. These researchers found African-American caregivers to be disproportionately female and poor. In addition, these caregivers were less educated and younger than their noncaregiving counterparts (Minkler & Fuller-Thomson). Despite the hardships implicated by these findings, African-American families continue to provide intergenerational kinship care.

It is no secret that African-American children, in general, face a number of challenges in the United States. For example, lower socioeconomic status and poor academic achievement have been demonstrated as impediments to successful life course outcomes for African-American children (for a review see Jencks & Phillips, 1998; Richman et al., 2004). Factors such as poverty, and the mental and physical health status of grandparent caregivers present additional challenges (Casper & Bryson, 1998). However, less evidence exists regarding how grandchildren achieve in school while being raised by their grandparent caregivers (Dench, 2002). Although the aforementioned factors present challenges for African-American children, education has been a key factor in negotiating various life stressors. Nurturing high expectations of academic achievement is a central value in the African-American community. As other researchers have confirmed, success is strongly linked to the social and family environments in which children are raised (Bradley, Corwyn, McAdoo, & Garcia Coll, 2001).

Likewise, social support is a crucial need for caregiving grandparents who often feel isolated and alienated in their parenting roles (Greene, 2006; Hayslip & Kaminski, 2005). Pruchno (1999) conducted one of the first large-scale studies to include both African-American and white grandmothers and found that African-American grandmothers were more likely than their white counterparts to have peers in close proximity also raising their grandchildren. Having a social support system provides grandparents an important outlet to share similar experiences. As with any group, a support network is vital for coping with the stressors that African-American custodial grandparents can experience.

Research Summary

The intergenerational literature mainly focuses on grandparents as kinship caregivers. Kinship care arrangements may be formal or informal, and provided by family relatives other than grandparents, though it is most commonly provided by grandparents (Brooks, Webster, Berrick, & Barth, 1998; Dubowitz, 1990; Simmons & Dye, 2003). Studies explicitly focused on the African-American family in the context of grandparent kinship caregivers and the education of their school-aged grandchildren, are sparse. That said, the kinship care literature may be consulted to inform this emerging and needed knowledge base.

School-related problems among youths in kinship and foster care have been consistently documented (Sawyer & Dubowitz, 1994; Seyfried, Pecora, Downs, Levine, & Emerson, 2000; Solomon & Marx, 1995); nevertheless, there is some evidence of school-related benefits for those children in kinship care placements (Dubowitz & Sawyer, 1994; Shin, 2003). For example, among 400 foster care youths in Illinois, Shin (2003) found a significant and positive relationship between kinship care placement and reading achievement scores: compared to adolescents in nonrelative placements, those in kinship care demonstrated significantly higher reading levels. On the basis of a sample of 374 children in kinship care, Dubowitz and Sawyer found better outcomes for kinship care youths on measures of school attendance, suspensions, and expulsion when compared to the general public school population in Baltimore, Maryland, despite their overall conclusion that children in kinship care exhibit school performance and behavior problems at higher rates than their classroom peers (Sawyer & Dubowitz, 1994).

When compared to counterparts in foster care and nonrelative placements, there is no empirical support for better outcomes among youth in kinship care on common outcome measures such as permanency placement (Courtney, 1994), behavior problems (Billing, Ehrle, & Kortenkamp, 2002; Eckenrode et al., 1993), and school problems (Billing et al., 2002; Eckenrode et al., 1993). Nonetheless, kinship care placements, both formal and informal, are increasingly a common practice for child welfare agencies (Child Welfare League of America, 1999; Crumbley & Little, 1997) and have been historically practiced within the African-American family (Fuller-Thomson & Minkler, 2000; McCullough-Chavis & Waites, 2004; Scannapieco & Jackson, 1996).

Theoretically, there are many advantages and benefits of kinship care for children including (1) placement with loving, caring, and familiar relatives whom children know and trust; (2) the reinforcement of family and cultural identity; and (3) family preservation (Cuddeback, 2004; Texas Department of Family and Protective Services, 2006). However, as observed by Cuddeback, "It is unknown if these advantages are more than theoretical, as few studies have explored these issues" (p. 634). It is imperative that this void in the literature be addressed because the theoretical advantages of kinship care highly characterize the cultural and historical reasons for which African-American families so frequently engage in intergenerational caregiving arrangements.

Although highly valued and commonly practiced in the African-American family, intergenerational caregiving presents many challenges for caregivers of school-aged children. Researchers have identified financial limitations, health issues, mental health status, caregiver burden, status of legal custody, and the *generation gap* as challenges faced by intergenerational caregivers (Burton, 1992; Fuller-Thomson & Minkler, 2000; Guzell-Roe, Gerard, & Landry-Meyer, 2005; Hill 2001; Morrow-Kondos, Weber, Cooper, & Hesser, 1997; Pruchno, 1999; Waldrop & Weber, 2001). For example, Lawrence-Webb, Okundaye, and Hafner (2003) conducted a qualitative study with nineteen African-American kinship caregivers of children with disabilities and identified education-related concerns in the following areas: (1) knowledge and understanding of the children's learning limitations and behavior problems; (2) assistance with modifying their parenting skills to adequately parent a new generation; and (3) improved home-school communication and outreach. In a comparative study of fourteen African-American and eleven Latino grandparent caregivers, Cox (2000) found African-American caregivers more likely to have legal guardianship and decision-making responsibilities for their grandchildren about counseling services, school, and camps.

Importantly, Strozier and colleagues' (2005) school-based intervention for seventy-two kinship caregivers (68 percent African American) of 235 children has implications for intergenerational influences on the education of African-American children. Their *Kinship Care Connection* intervention was designed to mediate caregiver burden in the areas of child behavior, self-advocacy, emotional support, school issues, and provider issues. Prior to the intervention, caregivers reported low levels of confidence in interacting with teachers and school administrators, which was perceived by school personnel as a lack of the caregivers' interest in the child. Post-test intervention measures of such behaviors revealed significant improvements among kinship caregivers, as well as in the areas of advocacy and emotional support (Strozier et al., 2005). Child participants also experienced significant overall improvements in self-esteem specific to home, school, and peers.

Owing to the small sample sizes, nonexperimental designs, and inconsistencies in differentiating grandparents from other kinship caregivers, these few studies cannot be generalized to the millions of African-American families who provide intergenerational caregiving. However, these studies do provide valuable insight into the issues faced by intergenerational African-American caregivers in educating children in their care, and offer directions for social work practice and future research in this area.

Examples of Intergenerational Programs That Address Educational Needs

In this section, we highlight two promising programs that have been implemented to enhance and support intergenerational caregiving with specific programmatic components that address the educational needs of children in these family structures: (1) the GrandFamilies House, and (2) the Project Healthy Grandparents (PHG) program.

The GrandFamilies House opened in 1999 in Boston, Massachusetts. This twenty-seven-unit facility houses grandparents who are raising their grandchildren and incorporates supportive enrichment services and interventions (Gelbspan & VanZandt, 1999). Three nonprofit agencies collaborated with the city and state to implement this program. One of the greatest challenges was securing a federally funded rent subsidy to provide funds for caregiving grandparents in need. Because most grandparents in the community were on fixed incomes, it was critical for the program developers to identify ways to subsidize the rent. After successfully securing funding, the Grand-Families House has become an affordable, supportive, and safe community for grandparents raising their grandchildren. On site, these families receive many social services such as legal assistance and counseling. Grandparents are able to attend support groups and psychoeducational groups designed specifically to meet their caregiving needs (e.g., parenting and behavior management). The children who reside at the GrandFamilies House may attend on-site preschool or receive after-school care and homework assistance, which is administered by the Boston YMCA. In addition, computer education is provided to the children and their grandparents. Not only are the services made available to the residents of GrandFamilies House, but they are available to other parenting grandparents also who live in the community and receive rent subsidies. The GrandFamilies model provides intergenerational families with social support as well as tangible support, both of which have been previously identified in this chapter as critical needs for this family structure.

The PHG began in 1995, at Georgia State University and has served more than 500 families and over 1,200 children. This strengths-based program provides a multitude of intervention services for grandparents who are raising their grandchildren (Perdue, 2006). A nationally recognized model, this intergenerational program brings together a cadre of professionals in the fields of social work, education, medicine, and allied health to engage custodial grandparents in addressing a multitude of stressors associated with caring for their grandchildren. Social workers conduct home visits and family assessments, and provide referrals to identified service providers for families to utilize. Registered nurses also conduct health assessments for grandparents with a focus on prevention and early intervention via health screenings such as cholesterol, blood pressure, diabetes, and vision.

An educational component of this program focuses on identifying grandchildren from ages zero to five years who may have developmental delays due to prenatal exposure to drugs and/or alcohol (Perdue, 2006). The PHG program collaborates with the Marcus Institute Fetal Alcohol Syndrome Clinic at Emory University to provide a comprehensive biopsychosocial and educational evaluation of the children in the program. Once the evaluations are completed, PHG works with the grandparents to implement any recommendations made as a result of the evaluations. Early intervention assessments such as this can influence the future educational experiences of the children because they prompt families to set early educational goals and to establish support systems, which are two of the strongest predictors of student development, motivation, academic success, college entry, and college aspirations (Tierney & Auerbach, 2004). In this regard, early intervention efforts can foster the transition to school, where school social workers can then cultivate and maintain the vital link between the school and family by engaging custodial grandparents and empowering them to assist and advocate for their grandchildren. In addition, a number of support services and parenting classes provide assistance to grandparents in this intergenerational family structure. PHG links families to support groups and other educational resources that aid in reducing the stress levels of these grandparents so that they in turn can help their grandchildren to thrive. Some of the support services that assist the grandparents in their new parenting roles include monthly parenting education classes, group counseling sessions, and transportation to participate in the services offered. This intergenerational project has been replicated within the University of Georgia system at three other campuses (University of Georgia, Valdosta State University, and the Medical College of Georgia) and nationally at three other universities, which include the University of Maryland-Baltimore, Winston-Salem State University, and Fordham University in New York. Each of these sites provides an enormous service to this growing population within their respective communities and helps build healthy families by empowering grandparent caregivers to succeed in parenting once again.

The programs described in this chapter can serve as models for how the educational needs of students living with grandparents can be addressed and supported. As this research knowledge base continues to develop, interventions such as these can inform social work practice with African-American intergenerational families. Given the increasing prevalence of this family structure, there will be adverse ramifications if their conditions and challenges go unaddressed. The implementation of more programs such as these has the potential to address the psychosocial and socioeconomic needs of African-American intergenerational families, and provide educational support for the children in their care, thereby improving educational outcomes for the next generation.

IMPLICATIONS FOR SCHOOL
SOCIAL WORK PRACTICE

School social workers are positioned and skillfully trained to facilitate family-school communication and collaboration that supports and assists grandparent caregivers and their school-aged grandchildren. Because of the adverse social conditions under which school-aged children may experience intergenerational kinship caregiving, school personnel and caregivers must understand the impact and implications of such occurrences on children's school experiences and educational performance. In this context, school social work roles, at the very least, include clinical interventionist, case manager, consultant, and diversity specialist (see Constable, Massat, McDonald, & Flynn, 2006).

As clinical interventionists with the children, school social workers should focus on addressing psychosocial needs. Greene (2006) recommends a solution-focused approach. Furthermore, a thorough, culturally sensitive and family systems-based assessment is required to screen for possible risk factors for academic problems (e.g., trauma, grief and loss, and behavior problems). Because of the potential for multiple issues that may exceed the capacity of school social workers, knowledge of relevant community resources and strong case management skills are imperative. A wraparound case management approach, with the school social worker as a primary source of information and referral, would be very beneficial to grandparent caregivers who often experience confusion and frustration when trying to navigate various systems to obtain services for their grandchildren (American Association of Retired Persons [AARP], 2003). As consultants and diversity specialists, school social workers are positioned to promote academic success for African-American children in intergenerational caregiving situations. Given their understanding of family systems theory, child development and cultural diversity, school social workers can help teachers and other school personnel better understand the needs of these students and heighten their awareness and "sensitivity to diversity in family structures" (Smith & Dannison, 2003, p. 51). In addition, school social workers can arrange mentoring relationships and tutoring services for such students when warranted and empower intergenerational caregivers to promote and support the children's education through psychoeducational sessions and support groups. Last, it is important for school social workers to address potential stereotypes of children in intergenerational care (Smith, Dannison, & Vach-Hasse, 1998) because teachers and school personnel may have negative assumptions about them (Rodriguez-Srednicki, 2002). For example, feelings of intimidation or refusal to disclose family secrets may be perceived by school personnel as resistance or a lack of interest on the part of caregivers (Cox, 2000; Strozier et al., 2005).

The complexity of this intergenerational family structure warrants intervention for the family system and the school as a system, at multiple ecological levels. Furthermore, school-based interventions with intergenerational African-American families should be implemented from a strengths perspective, given their strong cultural history of skipped- and three-generational kinship caregiving. Although research on the educational outcomes of students living with grandparents is sparse, there is some evidence that intergenerational kinship caregiving can be beneficial. Under the leadership of school social workers, school-based interventions that are family focused and culturally sensitive have great potential in promoting positive educational outcomes for African-American children in intergenerational caregiving families.

REFERENCES

Aldous, J. (1995). New views of grandparents in intergenerational context. *Journal of Family Issues, 16*(1), 104-123.

American Association of Retired Persons (AARP). (2003). *Lean on me: Support and minority outreach for grandparents raising grandchildren.* Washington, DC: Author. Retrieved May 25, 2006 from http://www.aarp.org/research/family/grandparenting/aresearch-import-483.html.

Barnes, S. L. (2001). Strengths and stressors: A theoretical and practical examination of nuclear, single-parent, and augmented African American families. *Families in Society: The Journal of Contemporary Human Services, 82*(5), 449-460.

Berrick, J. D., & Barth, R. P. (1991). The role of the school social worker in child abuse prevention. *Social Work in Education, 13,* 195-203.

Billing, A., Ehrle, J., & Kortenkamp, K. (2002). Children cared for by relatives: What do we know about their well-being? *New Federalism: National Survey of America's Families, Series B*(B-46). Washington, DC: Urban Institute. Retrieved November 14, 2007 from http://urbaninstitute.org/UploadedPDF/310486.pdf.

Bradley, R. H., Corwyn, R. F., McAdoo, H. P., & Garcia Coll, C. (2001). The home environments of children in the United States, Part 1: Variations by age, ethnicity, and poverty status. *Child Development, 72*(6), 1844-1867.

Brooks, D., Webster, D., Berrick, J. D., & Barth, R. P. (1998). *An overview of the child welfare system in California: Today's challenges and tomorrow's interventions.* Berkley, CA: Center for Social Service Research, University of California.

Brown, L. H. (2003). Intergenerational influences on perceptions of current relationships with grandparents. *Journal of Intergenerational Relationships, 1*(1), 95-111.

Bryson, K., & Casper, L. M. (1999). Coresident grandparents and grandparents. *Current Population Reports: Special Studies* (P23-198). Washington, DC: U.S.

Census Bureau, U.S. Department of Commerce, Economics and Statistics Administration. Retrieved June 1, 2006 from http://www.census.gov/prod/99pubs/p23198.pdf.

Burton, L. M. (1992). Black grandparents rearing children of drug-addicted parents: Stressors, outcomes, and social services needs. *Gerontologist, 32,* 744-751.

Carter, B., & McGoldrick, M. (Eds.) (2005). *The expanded family life cycle: Individual, family and social perspectives* (3rd ed.). Needham Heights, MA: Allyn & Bacon.

Casper, L., & Bryson, K. (1998). *Co-resident grandparents and their grandchildren: Grandparent maintained families* [Population Division Work Paper # 26]. Washington, DC: U.S. Bureau of the Census, Population Division. Retrieved June 22, 2006 from http://www.census.gov/population/www/documentation/twps0026/twps0026.html.

Child Welfare League of America. (1999). *CWLA standards of excellence for kinship care services.* Washington, DC: Author.

Constable, R., Massat, C. R., McDonald, S., & Flynn, J. P. (Eds.) (2006). *School social work: Practice, policy, and research* (6th ed.). Chicago: Lyceum Books.

Courtney, M. E. (1994). Factors associated with the reunification of foster children with their families. *Social Service Review, 68*(1), 81-108.

Cox, C. (2000). Empowering practice: Implications for interventions with African American and Latina custodial grandmothers. *Journal of Mental Health* and *Aging, 6*(4), 385-397.

Crumbley, J., & Little, R. L. (Eds.) (1997). *Relatives raising children: An overview of kinship care.* Washington, DC: Child Welfare League of America.

Cuddeback, G. S. (2004). Kinship family foster care: A methodological and substantive synthesis of research. *Children and Youth Services Review, 26,* 623-639.

Dench, G. (2002). *Grandmothers: The changing culture.* New Brunswick, NJ: Transaction Publishers.

Dubowitz, H. (1990). *The physical and mental health status of children placed with relatives: Final report.* Baltimore, MD: University of Maryland School of Medicine.

Dubowitz, H., & Sawyer, R. (1994). School behavior of children in kinship care. *Child Abuse and Neglect, 18,* 899-911.

Eckenrode, J., Laird, M., & Doris, J. (1993). School performance and disciplinary problems among abused and neglected children. *Developmental Psychology, 29*(1), 53-62.

Fuller-Thomson, E., & Minkler, M. (2000). African American grandparents raising grandchildren: A national profile of demographic and health characteristics. *Health and Social Work, 25*(2), 109-118.

Fuller-Thomson, E., Minkler, M., & Driver, D. (1997). A profile of grandparents raising grandchildren in the United States. *The Gerontologist, 37*(3), 406-411.

Gelbspan, A., & VanZandt, J. (1999, March). The GrandFamilies House. *Peacework Magazine* [online]. Retrieved June 16, 2006 from http://www.afc.org/pwork/0399/039902.htm.

Goodman, C., & Silverstein, M. (2002). Grandmothers raising grandchildren: Family structure and well-being in culturally diverse families. *The Gerontologist, 42*(5), 676-689.

Greene, R. R. (2006). Students living in the care of grandparents. In C. Franklin, M. B. Harris, & P. Allen-Meares (Eds.), *School services sourcebook: A guide for school-based professionals* (pp. 737-744). New York: Oxford University Press.

Guzell-Roe, J. R., Gerard, J. M., & Landry-Meyer, L. L. (2005). Custodial grandparents' perceived control over caregiving outcomes: Raising children the second time around. *Journal of Intergenerational Relationships, 3*(2), 43-61.

Hayslip, B. Jr., & Kaminski, P. (2005). Grandparents raising their grandchildren: A review of the literature and suggestions for practice. *The Gerontologist, 45*(2), 262-269.

Heywood, E. M. (1999). Custodial grandparents and their grandchildren. *The Family Journal: Counseling and Therapy for Couples and Families, 7*(4), 367-372.

Hill, T. (2001). What's a grandparent to do? The legal status of grandparents in the extended family. *Journal of Family Issues, 22*(5), 594-618.

Hunter, A., & Taylor, R. (1998). Grandparenthood in African American families. In M. Szinovacz (Ed.), *Handbook on grandparenthood* (pp. 70-86). Westport, CT: Greenwood Press.

Jencks, C., & Phillips, M. (Eds.) (1998). *The Black-White test score gap.* Washington, DC: Brookings Institution Press.

Lansford, J. E., Dodge, K. A., Pettit, G. S., Bates, J. E., Crozier, J., & Kaplow, J. (2002). A 12-year prospective study of the long-term effects of early child physical maltreatment on psychological, behavioral, and academic problems in adolescence. *Archives of Pediatrics and Adolescent Medicine, 156*(8), 824-830.

Lawrence-Webb, C., Okundaye, J. N., & Hafner, G. (2003). Education and kinship caregivers: Creating a new vision. *Families in Society: The Journal of Contemporary Human Services, 84*(1), 135-142.

Leach, M. T., & Williams, S. A. (In Press). The impact of the academic achievement gap on the African American family: A social inequality perspective. *Journal of Human Behavior in the Social Environment.*

McCullough-Chavis, A., & Waites, C. (2004). Genograms with African American families: Considering cultural context. *Journal of Family Social Work, 8*(2), 1-19.

Minkler, M. (1999). Intergenerational households headed by grandparents: Contexts, realities and implications for policy. *Journal of Aging Studies, 13*(2), 199-219.

Minkler, M., & Fuller-Thomson, E. (2005). African American grandparents raising grandchildren: A national study using the census 2000 American community survey. *Journal of Gerontology: Social Sciences, 60B*(2), S82-S92.

Morrow-Kondos, D., Weber, J. A., Cooper, K., & Hesser, J. L. (1997). Becoming parents again: Grandparents raising grandchildren. *Journal of Gerontological Social Work, 28*(1/2), 35-46.

Perdue, J. (2006). *Project healthy grandparents: Services.* Retrieved November 15, 2006 from http://www2.gsu.edu/~wwwalh/services.html.

Pruchno, R. (1999). Raising grandchildren: The experiences of black and white grandmothers. *The Gerontologist, 39*(2), 209-221.

Reynolds, G. P., Wright, J. V., & Beale, B. (2003). The roles of grandparents in educating today's children. *Journal of Instructional Psychology, 30*(4), 316-325.

Richman, J. M., Bowen, G. L., & Woolley, M. E. (2004). School failure: An eco-interactional developmental perspective. In M. W. Fraser (Ed.), *Risk and resilience in childhood: An ecological perspective* (2nd ed., pp. 133-160). Washington, DC: NASW Press.

Rodriguez-Srednicki, O. (2002). The custodial grandparent phenomenon: A challenge to schools and school psychology. *National Association of School Psychologists Communiqué, 31*(1). Retrieved June 19, 2006 from http://www.nasponline .org/futures/grandparents.html.

Ruiz, D. S., & Carlton-LaNey, I. (1999). The increase in intergenerational African American families headed by grandmothers. *Journal of Sociology and Social Welfare, 26*(4), 71-86.

Saluter, A. (1996). Marital status and living arrangements. *Current Population Reports Series.* Washington, DC: National Center for Health Statistics.

Sawyer, R., & Dubowitz, H. (1994). School performance of children in kinship care. *Child Abuse and Neglect, 18,* 587-597.

Scannapieco, M., & Jackson, S. (1996). Kinship care: The African American response to family preservation. *Social Work, 41*(2), 190-196.

Seyfried, S., Pecora, P., Downs, C., Levine, P., & Emerson, J. (2000). Assessing the educational outcomes of children in long-term foster care: First findings. *Journal of School Social Work, 24*(2), 68-88.

Shin, S. H. (2003). Building evidence to promote educational competence of youth in foster care. *Child Welfare, 82*(5), 615-632.

Simmons, T., & Dye, J. L. (2003). Grandparents living with grandchildren: 2000. *Census 2000 brief* (C2KBR-31). Washington, DC: U.S. Department of Commerce, Economic and Statistics Administration, U.S. Census Bureau. Retrieved May 30, 2006 from http://www.census.gov/prod/2003pubs/c2kbr-31.pdf.

Smith, A. B., & Dannison, L. L. (2003). Grandparent-headed families in the United States: Programming to meet unique needs. *Journal of Intergenerational Relationships, 1*(3), 35-47.

Smith, A. B., Dannison, L. L., & Vach-Hasse, R. (1998). When "grandma" is "mom": What today's teachers need to know. *Childhood Education, 75*(1), 12-16.

Solomon, J. C., & Marx, J. (1995). "To grandmother's house we go": Health and school adjustment of children raised solely by grandparents. *The Gerontologist, 35*(3), 386-394.

Strozier, A., McGrew, L., Krisman, K., & Smith, A. (2005). Kinship care connection: A school-based intervention for kinship caregivers and the children in their care. *Children and Youth Services Review, 27,* 1011-1029.

Texas Department of Family and Protective Services. (2006). *Kinship care.* Austin, TX: Author. Retrieved June 1, 2006 from http://www.dfps.state.tx.us/Child_ Protection/Kinship_Care/.

Tierney, W., & Auerbach, S. (2004). Toward developing an untapped resource: The role of families in college preparation. In W. Tierney, Z. Corwin, & J. Colyar (Eds.), *Preparing for college: Nine elements of effective outreach* (pp. 15-31). Albany, NY: State University of New York Press.

Turner, L. (1995). Grandparent-caregivers: Why parenting is different the second time around. *Family Resource Coalition Report, 14*(1-2), 6-7.

U.S. Senate. (1997). *Kinship Care Act of 1997* (S. 822). Washington, DC: Author. Retrieved June 15, 2006 from http://frwebgate.access.gpo.gov/cgibin/getdoc .cgi?dbname=105_ cong_bills&docid=f:s822is.txt.pdf.

Waldrop, D. P., & Weber, J. A. (2001). From grandparent to caregiver: The stress and satisfaction of raising grandchildren. *Families in Society: The Journal of Contemporary Human Services, 82*(5), 461-472.

Weber, J. A., & Waldrop, D. P. (2000). Grandparents raising grandchildren: Families in transition. *Journal of Gerontological Social Work, 33*(2), 27-46.

Chapter 8

Family Group Conferencing with African-American Families

Kilolo Brodie
Charnetta Gadling-Cole

Undoubtedly, the most enduring cultural strength that Black Americans brought with them from the African continent was the extended family and its strong kinship networks.

Hill, 1999, p. 123

Family group conferencing (FGC) is an intervention used by some practitioners in the helping profession (i.e., social workers and community liaisons) and human service agencies. The philosophical tenets of FGC support the aforementioned chapter quote regarding African-American families. FGC is a semiformal meeting that draws on the existing strengths that family members have and provides a context that mirrors the traditional values embodied in many African-American families. This chapter seeks to explore the relevance and cultural appropriateness of FGC as a tool for African-American families from an intergenerational standpoint.

In the recent past, FGC has been utilized as a mechanism to widen the circle of support around children in the foster care and juvenile justice systems. The authors propose that it can also be useful in providing long-term familial support to older adults and their network of caregivers. Through FGC, numerous intergenerational issues can be explored (i.e., housing, health care, child care, and education). FGC

Social Work Practice with African-American Families

has demonstrated its utility in public child welfare. This model of practice focuses on children and their families, but can be effective with older adults and the generation between them. The generation in between is often a caregiver, parent, adult child, or an extended family member. This middle-generation caregiver is likely to experience stress, besides, personal conflict and situational dilemmas. Therefore, an intergenerational approach is most beneficial in working with families, because each age cohort is threaded together and operates in concert with one another. This chapter will examine the informal supportive networks of African-American families, review some of the family-centered policies that have affected them, and provide theoretical perspectives that support FGC as a means to addressing the intergenerational needs of African Americans.

THE AFRICAN-AMERICAN HELPING EXPERIENCE AND FAMILY GROUP CONFERENCING

Historically, African-American families have always functioned in a pattern of sharing and exchange. The helping tradition was part of the African culture, prior to slavery (Miller, Randolph, Kaufman, Dargan, & Banks, 2000). One quality shared by nearly all African Americans was that life was organized around the family. In the present, "African American families continue to exist within the context of extended family structure rather than as discrete units. The members are interdependent and share [responsibilities]; members may share residences and/or resources to meet the needs of its members" (Stewart, 2004, p. 224). This tradition lends itself to family-centered approaches.

Numerous African Americans view family as a vital part of survival, as evidenced throughout the early historical experience of African people in the United States. This powerful ancestral lineage is the backbone and support for a number of African-American family systems. Working together as a holistic unit is an emphatic value of African culture/tradition and is often seen as a collective task among African Americans. At present, in many African-American families, individuals are conditioned to take on the task of supporting other family members who are experiencing difficulty. Family responsibility becomes an obligation that includes a variety of duties and roles, one being that of a caregiver.

In child welfare cases, using FGC with African-American families as a direct service practice strategy typically involves the identification of personal and professional networks that provide support to primary caregivers in meeting the emotional and developmental needs of children (Minnesota Department of Human Services, 2005). Caseworkers use the FGC practice modality once a case has been accepted and opened for case management services for the benefit of concurrent planning and expanding relative searches for potential child placements (Minnesota Department of Human Services, 2005). Another example of the applicability of family group conferences (FGCs) can be found in the plans that are generated from decision-making meetings. For instance, an FGC plan may dictate an uncle adapting his familial role with his niece/nephew into a more structured role (such as a formal mentor). In this example, the restructuring of family roles and positions are designed to aid the primary caregiver and provide needed guidance to the child(ren). Flexibility in familial roles is normative in African-American communities.

FGC and long-term care have two major points of intersection. Although long-term care comprises a myriad of services, it commonly refers to a system that provides social, personal, and health care services over a sustained period (ninety days or more) to people who suffer from chronic functional impairment (Barker, 1999; Garner, 1995). "Elderly people, most of whom are over age 75, are the primary recipients of long-term care" (Garner, 1995, p. 1629). FGCs can offer inherent benefits for an elder or an ill relative, as well as the primary caregiver. First, FGCs can be implemented to aid the caregiver in their, often heavy-laden, capacity. Adhering to the traditional African-American beliefs about the family unit, it is quite common for black families to choose to take care of older relatives in their own homes, rather than opting for a nursing home (Klopfenstein, 2001). FGCs require the family, as a whole, to decide how to address challenges even though only a few members may be directly affected.

Second, logistical plans that are focused on the physical care of an ailing family member are also appropriate for FGC. FGC plans can also incorporate ways to increase opportunities for social interaction for older adults in long-term care facilities, and establish respite for caregivers. Concrete, task-oriented plans of action provide explicit detail regarding what is needed, who is going to do it, and within a certain time frame. Planning for future outcomes is an essential part of an FGC.

AFRICAN-AMERICAN OLDER ADULTS, BABY BOOMERS, AND INTERGENERATIONAL CAREGIVING

Health Care and Older Adults

Inequity of access and underutilization of health services have contributed to the diminished health of the African-American older adult, which comprises the largest subgroup of older minority adults (Ford & Hatchett, 2001). African-American older adults when compared with Caucasian older adults are "more likely to be infirmed, to die (up to age eighty-five), to have chronic diseases at earlier ages and to be more physically limited by these illnesses" (Johnson, Gibson, & Luckey, 1990, p. 70). For the African-American older adult, poverty is frequently the result of lifelong patterns of discrimination and disadvantage (Miller et al., 2000). For the population of African-American older adults, the condition of poverty and/or substandard economic conditions often increase with age, thereby supporting the need for familial assistance and intergenerational caregiving.

Informal Support Systems

Informal or familial care of older adults, particularly African-American older adults, is the predominant form of older adult care (White-Means, 1993). According to Barresi and Menon (1990), "It is evident that the major sources of caregiving support for the African American elderly are their informal support networks. Both kin and nonkin networks provide for most African-American elderly's physical, psychological, and emotional needs" (p. 229). Informal caregiving is promoted within the African-American extended family system as it is an important resource for survival for its members (McAdoo, 1978; Scanzoni, 1977). African Americans of all ages are likely to live in an extended family household (Demo, Allen, & Fine, 2000). Extended family support is, therefore, important to both caregivers and older adults because many do not have sufficient financial resources to cope with [institutionalized] long-term care (Markides & Mindel, 1987).

Prior to the 1990s, informal support systems of the African-American aged, including both family and nonfamily supports, had been primary in the provision of services and supports to the African-American older adult (Barresi & Menon, 1990). Changes in population dynamics and the service delivery context, however, have impacted negatively on the family in its caregiving role, thus causing the informal support system of the African-American aged to weaken (Miller et al., 2000). FGC is a way of strengthening familial supportive networks and aiding those providing care to nuclear and extended relatives.

Baby Boomer Caregivers

Baby Boomers are likely to be the caregivers to the old and the caretakers of the young. According to American Association of Retired Persons (2001), African Americans represent 11 percent of the "sandwich" generation and face more potentially stressful situations than do members of other groups. AARP (2001) provides the following facts regarding African-American Baby Boomers: African-American Baby Boomers are particularly prone to enlist the support of their siblings and include them in their definition of family. Older African-American Baby Boomers are more inclined to take care of their parents or other relatives than are whites.

African Americans experience the highest incidence of potentially stress-inducing family and personal events, and suffer the highest probability of having had a family member die within the last year. In addition, African-American Baby Boomers are the most likely to have several children and expect children to assume filial responsibility that includes care of older adult family members as they age (Chavis & Waites, 2004). The coping mechanisms of African-American Baby Boomers frequently include religious faith, family connections, and their siblings (AARP, 2001) and adult children as caregivers (Chavis & Waites, 2004). These are essential elements that make FGC an appropriate tool for working holistically with family units and with multiple generations. The concept of collectivity and shared responsibility are fundamental to FGC and to the varied structural configuration of African-American families.

WHAT IS FAMILY GROUP CONFERENCING?

Family group conferencing (FGC) or family group conferences are semi-structured gatherings that recognize the value of extended family support, open up the lines of communication, and allow service providers and families to work together (Brodie & Gadling, 2004). FGCs integrate families into the decision-making process with regard to the well-being of their kin (Child Welfare Partnership/Portland State University, 2000). Family Group Decision Making (FGDM) is the overarching intervention strategy that encompasses FGC and similar versions of family meetings, such as team decision meetings, family unity meetings, structured team meetings, and so on.

The Historical Background of FGC

The origin of FGC is New Zealand, where it is practiced by the indigenous Maori people. In the 1970s and 1980s, Maori activists asserted themselves and sparked an interest in recapturing their culture by making efforts to receive compensation for their lost land at the hands of British colonists during the 1800s (Ernst, 1999; Fleras, 1995). This is similar to the Black Power movement that occurred in the United States in the 1960s and 1970s.

Shore, Wirth, Cahn, Yancey, and Gunderson (2002) define FGC as "a participatory approach to case planning that was originally developed by the Maori people of New Zealand, in response to concerns that the child welfare system was removing Maori children from their homes and cultural ties at a disproportionate rate" (p. 2). FGC ignited the importance of cultural identity in child protection policies and placed the onus of decision making on the family. This philosophy is also in concert with the thinking of many African-American families regarding the care of their own children. It may also be appropriate for intergenerational caregiving to aging family members.

Historically, kin have cared for children when parents were temporarily or permanently incapacitated (O'Brien, Massat, & Gleeson, 2001; Waites et al., 1999). In many cultures, such as the African-American culture, families still believe in relying on extended family support and community involvement. Conventional wisdom was the initial impetus driving FGC in the United States. At present, the scope of FGC spans across varied international populations. FGCs are being utilized in more than fourteen states in six countries worldwide (American Humane Association, 2003).

Since 1997, the American Humane Association—Children's Division has been at the forefront of FGC in child welfare (DiLorenzo, 2000). FGC builds on family strengths, rather than dwelling on family dysfunction, and provides the support needed to engage rather than alienate them (Pierce, 1999). The focus of social work on strengths-based, community-centered, and family-focused practice mirrors the tenets of family group conference. This family-centered approach can also work well in addressing family caregiving issues across the life span.

Phases of Family Group Conferencing

Referral. Typically, a service provider who is working with the family makes the referral for an FGC. Service providers can include, but are not limited to, social workers, community staff persons, attorneys, therapists, and other appropriate professionals. A referral is usually based on a perceived need by the service provider; however, family members can refer themselves.

Coordination. The coordinator's role includes ensuring the integrity of the process by interviewing all potential attendees. Participants usually include the child(ren)'s parents, extended family members, the family's significant close friends, and tribal elders (if appropriate) (American Humane Association, 1996). Some states conduct in-person interviews, usually in the form of a home visit to speak to relatives about the purpose of the FGC. Alternately, conversations about the process are held over telephone. Service providers are reminded by the coordinator of their particular role during the FGC, which is providing resources and helpers (Columbia Heights/Shaw Family Support Collaborative, 2001). Coordinators are expected to refrain from giving their opinions and recommendations regarding what decisions they believe that the family should make.

The coordinator is also responsible for logistics regarding location, time, desired meal to be served (chosen by the family), and daycare, if necessary. Travel arrangements, even for out of state or out of the country, are paid by the coordinator's agency. The time frame of an FGC meeting is from two to six hours, but typically lasts four hours.[1] The average time frame from referral to actually convening the FGC is approximately from twenty to forty hours (Burford, 2000; Nixon, Merkel-Holguin, Sivak, & Gunderson, 2000). The lengthy preparation time needed to coordinate an FGC helps ensure that it will be a qualitative and productive meeting.

The coordinator prepares a report for the facilitator describing the case history, interviews that were conducted, possible conflicts, and any nonnegotiable scenarios the agency might have faced. The final phase of coordination is usually completed within one week after the FGC. The coordinator is usually the one who types up the family's plan and hard copies are mailed to all who attended.

Facilitation. The facilitator usually receives a summary of the current situation and feedback from the interviews conducted by the coordinator. The report from the coordinator should provide the facilitator a semblance of the family's story. The gist of individual family members' challenges and triumphs, as well as a collective family history, should be evident (i.e., often outlined in a detailed genogram). The facilitator then devises his or her own strategies by identifying individuals who are potentially supportive and committed to the family, and those who may be antagonistic in the meeting or attempt to sabotage the plan. Attuned assessment skills and varied techniques are a prerequisite for a good facilitator. The facilitator keeps everyone on task according to the agenda. The facilitator needs to have had some aspect of formal family group conference training.

FGC Agenda. Families participating in an FGC are given the option of opening the meeting in their preferred conventional manner. The meeting typically begins with a culturally appropriate welcome according to the family's desires (i.e., prayer, moment of silence, etc.) (Connolly & McKenzie, 1999). Disclosures about mandated reporters in the room are mentioned and a consent form is circulated that needs to be signed by all the participants. In a narrative paragraph, the consent form outlines the participants' agreement to share information and to hold it in confidence so that it will not be used against anyone at a later date (primarily in court). After this segment of the FGC, all subsequent information is written down by the facilitator or cofacilitator on a flipchart to capture what is stated.

Goals are identified by the participants regarding what they hope to achieve from the FGC. Ground rules are established based on group norms (i.e., behaviors, attitudes, and perceptions that are approved of by the group and expected of its members) (Baron, Kerr, & Miller, 1992). Even though family members participate in setting the ground rules to guide the meeting they are not always implemented when practicing FGCs. The rationale is that the families can be trusted enough to work well without them, and it is one less authoritative procedure imposed onto the group.

Strengths and Concerns. Strengths and concerns/challenges is the next component of the conference. Strengths are those positive attributes that family members have individually or collectively. This is an opportunity for all of the participants to share what has been working well, and who has been an asset to the family or to the case itself. Emphasizing the strengths that families have is critical in being able to address the concerns. A creative, yet, stable plan can be developed and executed based on the positive qualities that are drawn. Concerns are issues that have caused difficulties for the family and/or service providers. During this phase of the FGC, participants explain to the group any reservations they might have, or obstacles that have limited progress.

Information Sharing. Information sharing is essential so that all participants can provide information to the group from their perspective. Families are afforded the opportunity to ask pertinent questions of those providing services to them. The facilitator also helps in framing and summarizing the critical issues presented before the group. Family members need the necessary information from service providers—void of the providers' personal opinions—for their decision-making process. Credentials are to be set aside during this phase of the FGC, and only the presentation of factual data is requested.

After the agency's bottom lines have been clarified and parameters for options established, the family meets alone. In the family's private discussion, all service providers exit the room and allow the family to deliberate as long as they need to generate a plan for the child(ren). There is no set limit on the length of time for the family to meet.

The entire group is reconvened when the family states that their meeting in private is over. Surprisingly to some, far more families have been able to make decisions about the care and protection of their children than not (Burford, 2000). The plans generated from these conferences are as good as or even better than they would have been without the family involvement (Burford, 2000). The plan is then presented to the service providers, who should fulfill any guidelines or legal requirements discussed during the information sharing session. Concrete details are elucidated to lessen the error when the plan is typed.

THEORETICAL FRAMEWORKS THAT SUPPORT FGC WITH AFRICAN-AMERICAN FAMILIES

The momentum of FGC has traversed into other nonchild welfare areas such as the school system, juvenile probation, adult protective services, and mental health (Challiner, Brown, & Lupton, 2000; Gunderson, 2000; Ordahl, Heinrichs, & Olmsted County Child and Family Services, 2000; Pennell & Burford, 1994, 1997, 2000). Subsequently, it has been proposed that other areas where FGCs are not yet prevalent, but could be used, are with African-American women as caregivers and caring for African-American older adults. A subtle consequence of ageism is the exclusion of older adults from participating in the production of knowledge about issues concerning them (Stewart, 2003). The older adults can contribute significantly, if they are given the opportunity to participate in decision making (Stewart, 2003). This is significant given the economic and health disparities faced by African-American older adults as well as their increasing life expectancy and overall numbers (Hooyman & Kiyak, 2005; Min, 2005). The implementation of FGC as a multigenerational perspective recognizes the importance of all generational linkages across the life span, including the important role of the middle generations and other cross-generational relationships (Fredriksen-Goldsen, Bonifas, & Hooyman, 2006).

Life Model

The life model is critical to understanding the theory underpinning FGC. Alex Gitterman (as cited in Turner, 1996) articulates the life model as a lens for viewing exchanges between people and their environments. Reciprocity among each other and between the communal environment is a common expectation for African-American families and their neighborhoods. FGC creates a physical context in the form of a group meeting that allows for the exchange of ideas between relatives and community service providers in a local milieu. Family group conferences are most often held in neutral places, such as community collaboratives, local centers, and so on. The life model examines relationships between living organisms and all the elements of the social and physical environments. The theoretical foundation for the life model is ecological theory.

Ecological Theory

To complement all the facets involved in FGC, a grounded theoretical framework is warranted. Factors that have contributed to the development of FGC include the environment at multiple levels (ecological perspective). The individuals and their social and physical surroundings are the focus when applying the ecological perspective. Amidst the varying age groups within the family, the individual in the middle generation is often burdened from providing assistance to older and younger family members (Carter & McGoldrick, 1999). For many African-American families, this is where reliance on other relatives and the immediate community come to the forefront. The extended family and how they socially affect or impact the ecological system is another theoretical angle that connects with the utility of FGC. The physical environmental context encompasses the entire structure of FGC.

Empowerment Perspective

The empowerment model is a theoretical perspective that is relevant to FGC as this model re-institutes power back into the hands of family members. This equal status relationship is optimized in a family group conference where the traditional professional hierarchy is shifted. Relatives are viewed equally responsible, if not more so, for generating viable outcomes that will work for their family. Elderly family members are often catalysts for gathering family members so that continuity of family functioning is maintained (Carter & McGoldrick,

1999). FGCs are designed to place ownership back into the hands of the family.

RELEVANT POLICY

Family-Centered Policy

A macrolevel shift from professionally centered models to family-centered models has unfolded. Dunst (1995) describes the differences between professionally centered and family-centered models. In professionally centered models families are viewed as incapable of solving their own problems; they are seen as deficient or pathological, requiring the expertise of professionals to function in a more healthier manner; and the professionals are characterized as experts who determine the needs of families from their own perspective instead of the family's perspective. In contrast, the five principles of a family-centered model are:

1. Enhance a sense of community
2. Mobilize resources and supports
3. Protect family integrity and strengthen family functioning
4. Share responsibility and collaborate
5. Adopt proactive program practices

These principles evoke empowerment, group decision making, and consumer-driven service delivery.

Family-centered services highlight the strengths of the family and its members as resources. An example of family-centered policy is Public Law 103-66. This legislation earmarked federal funds for family support and family preservation (McCrosky & Meezan, 1998). The family support/preservation legislation was designed to promote families' success, with funds allotted to assist with that goal. Public Law 103-66 also encouraged states to include the community in planning programs of child welfare agencies. Owing to lobbying and grassroots efforts, the government has allotted funds for family services, the encouragement of joint financial ventures between private and public entities, family-centered services, and an increased level of community involvement. Synthesis among local partnership and a multidisciplinary approach is evident during this era.

Public Policies and Older Adults

Practices and policies no longer fit the realities of a changing economy, changing gender roles, blurred lines between private and public roles, and a cohort of educated, introspective Baby Boomers newly valuing family life and uncertain about middle age. The beliefs about roles are inconsistent with the growing number of two-earner (or single-parent) Baby Boomer families as well as with the leading edge of these individuals moving into retirement. African-American Baby Boomers who are now in their late forties, fifties, and early sixties can expect to live well into their eighties and nineties. Although most older adults are active members of their families and communities, others need some type of assistance. Policies have been developed to address the needs of these individuals as discussed in the following section.

Americans with Disabilities Act

The public policies have been adopted directly and indirectly in the last fifteen years to address caregiver challenges. The Americans with Disabilities Act (ADA, 1990) has played a tremendous role in the enhancement of services for caregivers. Approximately 43 million Americans have one or more physical or mental disabilities; this number is increasing as the population continues to grow older (McArthur, 2001). Because incidents of disability increase dramatically after the age of sixty, the age groups with the highest proportion of people protected by the ADA are elders. Elderly and disabled individuals are highly susceptible to discrimination. The ADA is one policy that exists to assist this growing population toward more complete and integrated lives (McArthur, 2001) and at the same time providing the needed support for caregivers.

Service Provisions

In 1985, funding from the Older American's Act and the Community Care for the Elderly Act began the provision of services to sustain the impaired older person. The Community Care for Disabled

Adults funding was added to care for those persons eighteen years of age through fifty-nine years of age. This act is inclusive of multiple generations.

In response to caregiver stress, in 1992, states received appropriations from the Alzheimer's disease initiative respite care funds, which offers relief to the caregiver of an Alzheimer's victim. Major federal legislative, judicial, and administrative actions have affected state policies directly and indirectly changing the "landscape for family caregivers" (Fox-Grage, Coleman, & Blancato, 2001). These intergenerational policies include the following:

- In 1999, President Clinton unveiled his three-part long-term care plan. Two parts are enacted: The National Family Caregiver Support Program and the Long-Term Care Security Act. The tax credit for family caregivers was passed in 2001 as part of the Long-Term Care and Retirement Security Act of 2001.
- The settlements reached by the state attorney general and the tobacco industry in the late 1990s has created a new source of revenue for home and community-based care services and respite care (Fox-Grage et al., 2001).

National Caregiver Initiative

The Older Americans Act Amendments of 2000 (Public Law 106-501) established an important new program, the National Family Caregiver Support Program (NFCSP). Caregivers are finally receiving recognition for the services they provide that not only benefits their care recipient, but also provides tremendous economic relief to society.

PRACTICE IMPLICATIONS

Social workers who work with older adults often collaborate with extended family members (i.e., for long-term planning of the aged, coordinating visitation schedules, authorization of their medical care, etc.). Social workers can play a key role in fostering effective involvement with family members across the long-term care continuum (Gaugler, Anderson, & Leach, 2003). On the other side of the spectrum, social workers who work with children regularly have to engage the youths' familial network for kinship placements (i.e., grandparents as the caretakers), parental authorization for activities and services, arrangement of visitation schedules, and so on. Depending on the social work setting, FGC can easily be an appropriate method for including multiple generations in problem solving and inclusive decision making. Elders' participation in decision making is valuable (Stewart, 2003). The advanced skills of an FGC coordinator and facilitator include the ability to encourage participants and to clarify and summarize information; these elements are essential when working with older populations (Stewart, 2003). Social work practice with the young and the old is often not done in isolation of one another. A multigenerational approach through FGC can help social work professionals work within, as well as across, generations (Fredriksen-Goldsen, Bonifas, & Hooyman, 2006).

"Family group decision making fits well within cultures that have strong family bonds. . . ." (Welty, 1997, p. 4). Some may argue that trained professionals should be the ones to make decisions for children, female caregivers, and the aged. There are service providers who are concerned that general safety and well-being may be compromised if the decision-making role is turned over to the family. Many fear that families do not have the ability to make difficult decisions about what is best. "According to anthropological and ethnographic research, many of the resiliency-producing values and successful coping strategies of contemporary Black families are cultural strengths that are derived from their African legacy" (Hill, 1999, p. 149). The notion that this is no longer possible gets challenged from time to time. Anecdotal reports, however, indicate that families often come up with more creative and thoughtful plans than trained professionals (Welty, 1997).

If service providers want to harness the cultural strengths of the family and its community support system, the providers must recognize and appreciate the values, traditions, and history of that family's community (Connolly & McKenzie, 1999). "Awareness of one's own values, assumptions, and behaviors is necessary for developing the skills that facilitate empathic interaction with clients and appreciation of culturally different others" (Pinderhughes, 1989, p. 20). To do this "requires an in-depth understanding of one's own cultural background and its meaning" (Pinderhughes, p. 20). Personal exploration is imperative in order to avoid or minimize the projection of a potentially disheartened attitude and the possible promotion of negative perceptions when working with families.

CONCLUSIONS AND RECOMMENDATIONS

"In order for family-based interventions to have the greatest impact in routine practice, social workers should be involved in administering staff-family contacts and relationships, mediating any potential conflicts that occur between staff and family members. . . ." (Gaugler, Anderson, & Leach, 2003, p. 25). This challenge can be achieved through thorough FGC coordination and facilitation. Multiple levels of family participation and conflict resolution should be the focus of social work practitioners.

According to Stewart (2003), researchers have not extended sufficient opportunities to older adults so that their voices can be heard. Perhaps soliciting input from the aged should be the focus of more social work researchers. The implementation of FGC would help to address this concern by incorporating elders throughout the entire process. The older adult would be included at the onset of preparing for an FGC through solution-focused interviewing techniques, the facilitated meeting itself, and the follow-up plan delineating subsequent actions of relatives and service providers. More researched documentation on FGCs with this particular population is needed.

Although FGCs support the innate functions within black families (i.e., collectivity, community support, reliance on kin),

> [it] must acknowledged that no model can hope to fit and accommodate the needs of all families. The challenge is to find a process of best practice that is sensitive to differences and is sufficiently flexible to adapt to diverse needs and demands. (Connolly & McKenzie, 1999, p. 68)

FGC does show promises as a tool for African-American families from an intergenerational standpoint. This model can be used to build on family resilience and solidarity.

NOTE

1. This information was gathered from Columbia Heights/Shaw Family Support Collaborative in Washington, DC.

REFERENCES

American Association of Retired Persons (AARP). (2002). *In the middle: A report on multicultural boomers coping with family and aging issues.* Available online: http://research.aarp.org/il/in_the_middle_1.html.

American Humane Association. (2003). *FGDM programs around the world.* Retrieved March 16, 2003 from http://www.americanhumane.org/fgdm/projects.asp.

American Humane Association. (1996). Family group decision making: A promising new approach for child welfare. *Child Protection Leader,* July, p. 4.

Barker, R. (1999). *Social work dictionary.* Washington, DC: NASW Press.

Baron, R. S., Kerr, N. L., & Miller, N. (1992). *Group process, group decision, group action.* Bristol, PA: Open University Press.

Barresi, C. M., & Menon, G. (1990). Diversity in black family caregiving. In Z. Harel, E. A. McKinney, & M. Williams (Eds.), *Black aged: Understanding diversity and service needs* (pp. 221-235). Newbury Park, CA: Sage.

Brodie, K., & Gadling, C. (2003). The use of family decision meetings when addressing caregiver stress. *Journal of Gerontological Social Work, 42*(1), 89-100.

Burford, G. (2000). Advancing innovations: Family group decision making as community-centered child and family work. *Protecting Children, 16*(3), 3.

Carter, B., & McGoldrick, M. (1999). *The expanded family life cycle: Individual, family, and social perspectives* (3rd ed.). Needham Heights, MA: Allyn & Bacon.

Challiner, V., Brown, L., & Lupton, C. (2000). A survey of family group conference use across England and Wales. In the *National Roundtable on Family Group Decision Making: Summary of Proceedings* in Madison, WI. Englewood, CO: American Humane Association.

Chavis, A., & Waites, C. (2004). Genograms with African American families: Considering cultural context. *Journal of Family Social Work, 8,* 2.

Child Welfare Partnership, Portland State University. (July, 2000). *Family decision meetings: A profile of average use in Oregon's child welfare agency—final report.* Retrieved January 12, 2001 from http://www.ahafgdm.org/research/finalrep.

Columbia Heights/Shaw Family Support Collaborative. (2001). *Family group conferencing overview.* Training Manual. Washington, DC.

Connolly, M., & McKenzie, M. (1999). *Effective participatory practice: Family group conference in child protection.* Hawthorne, NY: Aldine De Gruyter.

Demo, D. H., Allen, K. R., & Fine, M. A. (Eds.) (2000). *Handbook of family diversity.* New York: Oxford University Press.

DiLorenzo, P. (2000). Family group decision making: A circle of support. *Protecting Children, 16*(3), 3.

Dunst, C. (1995). *Key characteristics and features of community-based family support programs.* Chicago, IL: Family Resource Coalition, Best practices Project.

Ernst, J. S. (1999). Whanau knows best: Kinship care in New Zealand. In R. L. Hegar, & M. Scannapieco (Eds.), *Child welfare: A series in child welfare practice, policy, and research.* New York: Oxford University Press.

Fleras, A. J. (1995). From social welfare to community development: Maori policy and the department of Maori affairs in New Zealand. In J. Rothman, J. L. Erlich, & J. E. Tropman (Eds.), *Strategies of community intervention* (5th ed.). Itasca, IL: F. E. Peacock Publishers.

Ford, M. E., & Hatchett, B. (2001). Gerontological social work with older African American adults. *Journal of Gerontological Social Work, 36,* 141-55.

Fox-Grage, W., Coleman, B., & Blancato, R. B. (2001). *Federal and state policy in family caregiving: Recent victories but uncertain future.* San Francisco: Family Caregiver Alliance.

Fredriksen-Goldsen, K. I., Bonifas, R. P., & Hooyman, N. R. (2006). Multigenerational practice: An innovative infusion approach. *Journal of Social Work Education, 42*(1), 25-36.

Garner, J. D. (1995). Long-term care. In R. L. Edwards & J. G. Hopps (Eds.), *Encyclopedia of social work* (19th ed.). Washington, DC: NASW Press.

Gaugler, J. E., Anderson, K. A., & Leach, C. R. (2003). Predictors of family involvement in residential long-term care. *Journal of Gerontological Social Work, 42*(1), 3-26.

Gunderson, J. (2000). The family group conference: An innovative approach to truancy in schools. In the *National Roundtable on Family Group Decision Making: Summary of Proceedings* in Madison, WI. Englewood, CO: American Humane Association.

Hill, R. (1999). *The strengths of African American families twenty-five years later.* Lanham, MD: University Press of America.

Hooyman, N., & Kiyak, H. A. (2005). *Social gerontology: A multidisciplinary perspective.* Boston: Allyn & Bacon.

Johnson, H. R., Gibson, R. C., & Luckey, I. (1990). *Health and social characteristics: Implications for services* (pp. 69-81). Newbury Park, CA: Sage.

Klopfenstein, S. (2001). Few blacks in county nursing homes. *The Journal Star,* July, 25.

Markides, K. S., & Mindel, C. H. (1987). *Aging and ethnicity.* Sage Library of Social Research, 163. Newberry Park, NJ: Sage.

McAdoo, H. P. (1978). Factors related to stability in upwardly mobile black families. *Journal of Marriage and the Family, 40*(4), 761-776.

McArthur, D. (2001). *Americans with Disabilities Act of 1990 and Accessibility of State and Local Court Facilities, Programs, and Services.* Available online: http://www.keln.org/bibs/mcarthur.html#IV.

McCroskey, J., & Meezan, W. (1998). Family-centered services: Approaches and effectiveness. *Protecting Children from Abuse and Neglect, 8*(1), 6.

Miller, R., Randolph, S., Kaufman, C., Dargan, V., & Banks, D. (2000). *Non-family caregivers of the African American elderly: Research needs and issues.* Available online: http://www.rcgd.isr.umich.edu/prba/perspectives/springsummer2000/srandolp2.pdf.

Min, J. W. (2005). Culturally competency: A key to effective future social work with racially and ethnically divers elders. *Families in Society: The Journal of Contemporary Social Services, 86*(3), 347-358.

Minnesota Department of Human Services. (2005). *The role of the caseworker in identifying, developing and supporting strengths in African American families involved in child protective services: A practice guide.* Available online: www.dhs.state.mn.us.

Nixon, P., Merkel-Holguin, L., Sivak, P., & Gunderson, K. (2000). How can family group conferences become family-driven? Some dilemmas and possibilities. *Protecting Children, 16*(3), 3.

O'Brien, P., Massat, C. R., & Gleeson, J. P. (2001). Upping the ante: Relative caregivers' perceptions of changes in child welfare policies. *Child Welfare, 80*(6), 719-748.

Ordahl, T. L., Heinrichs, M., & Olmsted County Child and Family Services. (2000). In the *National Roundtable on Family Group Decision Making: Summary of Proceedings* in Madison, WI. Englewood, CO: American Humane Association.

Pennell, J., & Burford, G. (1994). Widening the circle: Family group decision making. *Journal of Child and Youth Care, 9*(1), 1-11.

Pennell, J., & Burford, G. (1997). The family group making project: Communities of concern for resolving child and adult abuse. In G. Burford (Ed.), *Ties that bind: An anthology of social work and social welfare in Newfoundland and Labrador* (pp. 280-289). St. John's, NF: Jesperson.

Pennell, J., & Burford, G. (2000). Family group decision making: Protecting women and children. *Child Welfare, 79*(2), 131-158.

Pierce, L. (1999). Kinship foster care: Policy, practice, and research. *Families in Society: The Journal of Contemporary Social Services, 80*(4), 423-425.

Pinderhughes, E. (1989). *Understanding race, ethnicity, and power: The key to effective clinical practice.* New York: Free Press.

Scanzoni, J. (1979). Changing sex roles and emerging directions in family decision making. *Journal of Consumer Research, 4*(3), 185-188.

Shore, N., Wirth, J., Cahn, K., Yancey, B., & Gunderson, K. (2001). *Long-term and immediate outcomes of family group conferencing in Washington state.* Retrieved February 6, 2002 from http://www.ahafgdm.org/research.

Stewart, P. E. (2004). Afrocentric approaches to working with African American families. *Families in Society: The Journal of Contemporary Social Services, 85*(2), 221-228.

Stewart, S. (2003). A tapestry of voices: Using elder focus groups to guide applied research practice. *Journal of Gerontological Social Work, 42*(1), 77-88.

Turner, F. J. (1996). *Social work treatment* (4th ed.). New York: Free Press.

Waites, C., Macgowan, M., Pennell, J., & Weil, M. (1999). Family group conferencing: Building partnerships with African American, Latino/Hispanos, and American

Indian families and communities. *Family Group Decision Making Roundtable Proceedings*. Englewood, CO: American Humane Association.

Welty, K. (1997). *Family group decision making: Implications for permanency planning*. North American Council on Adoptable Children (NACAC).

White-Means, S. I. (1993). Informal home care for frail black elderly. *Journal of Applied Gerontology, 12*(1), 18-33.

Chapter 9

Intergenerational Caregiving: Family and Long-Term Care

Molly Everett Davis
Cheryl Waites

It's a labor of love, but it exacts a tremendous toll from people who have few resources to begin with.

New York Times on the Web

There is a long tradition of caregiving within the African-American community. The culture of caregiving is intergenerational in nature and has existed within an informal community context. Even today, caregiving in African-American families is intergenerational in nature. African-American caregivers are more likely to have children under age eighteen living in the household than caregivers from other racial or ethnic groups. This suggests a prevalence of intergenerational caregiving—caring for both the younger and older generations simultaneously.

Caregiving in the African-American family is based on a sense of common history and connection that has helped the family to survive oppression and injustice. Family support and kinship networks have been critical to the survival of the black community. This tradition may have stemmed from the culture and traditions that existed in African villages. It could have also evolved from life in the slave quarters of the plantations when it was obvious slaves could not count on the master's benevolence in times of need.

Social Work Practice with African-American Families

This chapter examines intergenerational support and caregiving as it pertains to patterns of exchange between elder African Americans and their families. The traditions of family caregiving also have important implications for long-term care of African Americans. The characteristics of intergenerational relations pertaining to family caregiving and elders who reside in long-term care facilities are also discussed.

INTERGENERATIONAL RELATIONSHIPS AND CAREGIVING

The notion of intergenerational relationships is vital to an understanding of caregiving in the African-American family. Intergenerational relationships are a qualitative measure of the connection among members of the family in different age groups. There are continuing transfers between different generations to support caregiving and relationships, ranging from young caregivers taking care of adults to adult caregivers providing kinship care for the family.

African-American families have been able to transfer across generations a sense of commitment, responsibility, and connection that has served to strengthen the bonds of intergenerational relationships. A strong tradition of "taking care of each other" evolved as a coping strategy against an oppressive dominant culture. There are several perspectives on why social support is extended within families and across generations to facilitate exchange of resources. The theories that follow provide a framework for understanding these bonds.

Theories

Attachment theory (Bowlby, 1988) suggests that the strength of early relationships form a persistent pattern of closeness that facilitates social exchange over time. Strong early positive relationships provide a foundation for lifelong reciprocal relationships that provide continuity. Social support is a product of high quality, early persistent relationships, and historical lifeways that promote a willingness to engage in caregiving roles.

The Support Bank theory (Antonucci, 1991) suggests lifelong exchanges and caregiving can be represented through the processes of investment and withdrawal over time. Parents begin investing in the support bank during the early years of the life cycle. This investment in children is available later for withdrawal by the elderly parent. Over the lifetime the exchanges may not be equal or reciprocal but over time it generationally achieves greater balance. These theories seek to provide a rationale for the caregiving over a lifetime that can be observed in African-American families and other ethnic groups as well. This pattern or dynamic is heavily tied into traditions and rituals that are a strong part of the cultural heritage of African Americans.

The term *intergenerational solidarity* refers to the quality and character of relationships that exist across generations. This term is particularly important in understanding the changes that have occurred qualitatively in the nature of intergenerational relationships within the African-American family over time. As a social unit, the African-American family has been impacted by changes in family roles, relationships, institutional policies, and programs.

It is important that there be an understanding of how intergenerational relationships stem from historical patterns and lifeways but change or adapt in the context of family and environmental demands. Intergenerational relationships are usually explored in three main areas: (1) emotional closeness; (2) amount of contact and physical proximity across generations; and (3) directional exchange of resources and social support. These areas are closely related to the nature and character of caregiving experiences within the African-American family.

CAREGIVING
IN THE AFRICAN-AMERICAN FAMILY

In the African-American community intergenerational family caregiving is commonly observed. African Americans often rely heavily on family members as a primary source of support (Dilworth-Anderson, Williams, & Gibson, 2002). There are 22.4 million caregiving households in America. More than 10 percent of these households are African Americans (www.marketsearch.com). African-American caregivers spend on average twenty-one hours per week providing care to children or dependent elders. Even though a large number of African Americans provide caregiving, 66 percent of them are employed full- or part-time (www.seniorhealth.about.com).

The norm within most African-American families is that children should take care of their older family members. There is a long-standing tradition of valuing elders that has a foundation in the faith or religious teachings of African Americans (Moody, 1996). Caregiving also extends to children when adult children are not able to do so. Those who provide kinship care are more likely to be older, single, financially unstable, less educated, and African American when compared with all foster caregivers (Berrick, 1998; Courtney & Needell, 1997; Ehrle & Geen, 2002). This cultural value of caregiving has been passed on to each successive generation.

Ongoing exchange of support, when needed, seems connected to strong attachment bonds and to respecting family values, traditions, and obligations (Taylor, 1985; Taylor, Chatters, & Jackson, 1997). Family members provide material support to meet the needs of elder family members and in return, the elders are able to provide advice and counsel in resolving family issues. Elders serve as the core on which the family network remains connected. Kopera-Frye and Wiscott (2000) describe the role of African-American grandparents as "keepers of culture." This exchange of support, reciprocity, and mutual aid represents an intergenerational pattern designed to facilitate respect, reverence, and open communication across generations. These intergenerational relationships provide life direction, advice, teachings on interpersonal relationship, religion, and values (Kopera-Frye & Wiscott, 2000; Strom, Collingsworth, Strom, & Griswold, 1993).

Caregiving in the African-American family is a testament to its resilience and strengths. Because African-American caregivers tend to have less financial resources, caregiving places a disproportionate amount of strain on the caregiver. African-American caregivers when compared with whites are more likely to say that caregiving is a financial hardship—22 percent as compared to 10 percent for whites (National Alliance for Caregiving and AARP, 2004). This is reflected in the following excerpt.

The doorbell rang and ten-year-old Bernard rushed to see who was at the door. His grandmother, Jennie from the bedroom called for him to be careful and always ask for the name before opening the door. Bernard asked the stranger who was calling and the woman announced that she was the school social worker from Watley Elementary school. The social worker asked if she could come in. After receiving permission from his grandmother, Bernard opened the door. The social worker indicated that Bernard had been absent from school over fifty days and she was concerned that he would be significantly behind his peers because of his absenteeism. She reminded the older woman that there are laws about school attendance. Grandmother Jennie felt bad. She had agreed to take care of her grandson after his parents became ill with HIV/AIDS. She had had to keep Bernard home on days whenever she had difficulty getting out of bed because of a chronic illness. He was a good helper and she did not know how she would have made it without his help. Although the social worker understood the plight of Grandma Jennie, Bernard would be in severe trouble if he continues to miss his attendance.

Caregiving is a complex issue in contemporary practice. African-American caregivers often find themselves caught between what is possible and what they are obligated to do. The vignette depicts a young caregiver with responsibilities to his grandmother. The demands of caregiving, although a part of the cultural tradition within the African-American family, can be very stressful and increasingly difficult without support and assistance. The caregiving experience of many older African Americans is associated with both social isolation and economic hardships (O'Brien, Massat, & Gleeson, 2001). There is a great deal of stress and burden associated with the caregiving experience, including challenges to health and well-being (Minkler, Roe, & Price, 1992). Caregiving grandparents are more likely to have depressive symptoms when compared to noncaregiving grandparents (Fuller-Thompson & Minkler, 2000). Schulz and Beach (1999) found that elderly caregiving spouses who report experiencing strain have a greater risk of death than those who are not caregivers. Their research suggests a 63 percent higher risk of death than noncaregivers. The significance of social support both formal and informal has been documented (Dilworth-Anderson et al., 2002). Yet, African-American families are less likely to use formal support as family members' physical limitation and needs increase.

FAMILY CAREGIVING TRADITIONS

Caregiving is a tradition with a long-standing history in the African-American family. The idea represented in the African proverb, "It takes a village to raise a child," reflects the expressed community concern for taking care of each other. African-American families prefer to care for elders in their homes when feasible. This preference is based on a culture that supports informal care, a belief that "one should take care of your own family" and a distrust of formal caregiving organizations. Underutilization of formal services is a well-established fact for African Americans (Cagney & Agree, 1999).

Some caregiving, however, is more related to the realities of being an oppressed people unable to access caregiving resources available to dominant groups. This practice of caregiving should not be utilized as a means to rationalize denial of care to African-American families. In many aspects, the preference for care in the home and underutilization of formal supports (long-term care, respite, etc.) may be linked to segregation, economic disparities, and barriers to access.

Caregiving is a substantial issue in the African-American family. As is true with many other groups, women are the primary providers of caregiving (Spector, 2000). In fact, the increased participation of women in the workforce is believed to be a factor in greater utilization of formal long-term services (Callahan, 1996). African-American caregivers are more likely to live with the recipients of this care (Mutran, 1985). Carlton-LaNey (2006) outlines an African-American caregiving paradigm that is prevalent in rural communities. She reports a reliance on informal and communal resources such as church elders, stewards, deacon, and secret orders such as the Masons and Eastern Star, natural or faith healers, general stores, and home demonstration clubs. There is an increasing trend toward substituting formal for informal services when these services are available, accessible, and affordable (National Alliance for Caregiving and AARP, 2004, Met Life Study).

Family Caregiving—An Ethic of Responsibility. The concept of filial responsibility should be examined to understand the roots of caregiving in the African-American family. It illustrates the perceived responsibility that adult children have to aged parents in regard to care and assistance (Bonner, Gorelick, & Prohaska, 1999). In fact, some references call it *filial obligation because of its importance to family life.* Filial responsibility is a term that demonstrates a resilience of family relationships for information exchange.

The term functional solidarity (discussed in Chapter 2) is also related to the concept of filial responsibility and refers to the exchange of assistance between generations (Bengtson & Robert, 1991). It focuses on the core of family relationships and the ways in which connections are made within families. Filial obligation is strong among African-American caregivers (Pinquart & Sorensen, 2005). The expectation of care is traditionally at the heart of those seeking caregiving that is prevalent in African-American families.

Variations in Caregiving. Multiple kinds of caregiving exist within African-American families and the network of kinship relationships. As discussed in this chapter (and book) children may reside with caregiving relatives without formal foster care or adoption processes. Children may also care for parents and older or disabled relatives. Caregiving includes kinship care or relatives raising children, inter-generational coresidence, young caregivers for the disabled and in-firm as well as care for elders who are in long-term care facilities. These informal relationships have historically been characteristic of the kinship relationships that exist within the black family.

Although there has been a long-standing history of reliance upon the family system to support African-American elders and family caregiving, there are differences with every generation. This is due to cohort effects. *Cohort* refers to the norms, beliefs, values, and the historical influences that shape each generation. Cohorts of people not only share the experience of certain life events, but they also develop specific *lifeways* as a result of these experiences. *Lifeways* are adaptive responses reflected in traditions, rituals, behavior patterns, and customs. For example, many individuals who lived during the Depression had similar lifeways. These lifeways are often characterized by frugality, distrust of banks, and a greater propensity to save money. When the cohort of older adults who lived during the Depression is compared to Baby Boomers who are beginning to enter old age, significant differences in lifeways are observable.

The second factor is related to the development of and access to institutional social programs that are designed to address and meet family needs. The increased reliance of African Americans on social welfare services has led to reduced expectation of families to provide frontline care to family members. Government is often viewed as the provider of goods and services for older adults and families continue to play supportive roles.

Intergenerational Conflict

Family relationships have a history and they change over time. Intergenerational conflict can occur when there are generational cohort differences. History within families often crosses generations and may lead to intergenerational conflict. The term "filial crisis" represents the idea that parent-child conflicts that begin in adolescence often continue into later life. The underlying concept is that long-term, complex, family problems and unresolved conflicts that influence family relations can impact the treatment of older adults (Godkin, Wolf, & Pillemer, 1989).

African-American families experience this dynamic concept. It cannot be assumed that because of the culture of caring that existed in African-American families, intergenerational conflict will not occur. In addition, there is varying consensus within families concerning their responsibility to take care of older adult family members. Some family members feel this responsibility more strongly than others. It would be a mistake to assume that there is uniformity in perspectives. The following example illustrates a relationship in which there is a history of conflict influencing the mother/daughter relationship, after the mother's admission to a nursing home:

Jean and her mother were always in conflict. Mrs. Brown felt that Jean was the only one of her children who gave her problems. She always made comparisons of Jean with her siblings. Over the years there was continued conflict between Jean and her mother. They would only see each other once in a year and eventually there would be an argument. Jean was the only sibling living in the same town when Mrs. Brown could no longer live alone and needed nursing home care. Although she visited her mother during the first week of her stay in the nursing home, the staff witnessed an argument between the two. Jean has not returned for the last three months.

African-American families have different attachment bonds owing to a number of factors. African-American families have been impacted by many of the same forces that have touched families in the dominant culture. Family violence, trauma, substance abuse, and dysfunctional patterns in families inhibit strong attachment bonds (Hummert & Morgan, 2001). The increasing numbers of divorces, blended families, and cohabiting couples create family fragmentation and significantly enlarge the family network, sometimes beyond the ability to sustain contact and relationship (Clarke, Preston, Raskin, & Bengtson, 1999). Also, patterns of employment that increase the geographic distances among family members have impacted attachment bonds (Ingersoll-Dayton, Neal, & Hammer, 2001). It is not uncommon that younger family members have little or no contact with older family members. This detachment of relationships can ultimately impact the older adult when assistance or support is required.

Health Issues and Caregiving

African-American elders often do not complain (Carlton-LaNey, 2006). The mere fact that the older adult has survived into old age is viewed with gratitude. They are less likely to seek health care early and more likely to rate their health as poor (Adams & Jackson, 2000). Many African-American elders have knowledge of folk medicine techniques that they often employ to help themselves and their families in the home setting (Baer & Merrill, 1981; Baer & Nichols, 2001). Many folk remedies and attitudes about illnesses are reinforced through intergenerational transmissions. Sometimes, the visits to the doctors in the hospital could be only long after it is clear that the traditional practices are not working.

African-American elders often have chronic health problems as a result of many factors, including the lack of preventive health care. Many chronic health conditions (hypertension, diabetes, and chronic heart condition) lead to disability and the need for assistance from family and sometimes placement in long-term care facilities. In the past, African-American elders used nursing homes for rehabilitation. Traditionally, lower rates of nursing home care (and long-term care placement as a whole) were associated with home-based caregiving, Medicaid discrimination, and the lack of available beds at the federal/state level (Mavundia, 1996). Within the last few years, the pattern of nursing home utilization by African Americans has changed. Nursing home utilization is currently equal to or greater than that of white Americans (National Center for Health Statistics, 1999).

CAREGIVING AND LONG-TERM CARE

Elders are usually moved to health care facilities or long-term care facilities (nursing homes) as residents owing to a decreasing health status or a traumatic event such as a fall or accident. Family caregivers are determined that they need formal assistance for the care of their elder relative. Often, this is a difficult decision for family members. In some cases, there may be no family member who can physically or financially provide informal care. Because of a strong tradition of caregiving in the African-American family, guilt and shame may be associated with placement into a long-term care facility, especially for those who are older adults.

For African Americans born before 1935, the nursing home in their youth was referred to as "old folks home." In most communities, this facility existed and was usually reserved for frail older adults and those who had no family. The perception of the facility was usually negative. Residing in such a facility meant that there was no family member available to help in old age. There was also a fear that one might be maltreated in some form or used for experiments without consent, such as in the Tuskegee project. All of these factors contribute to anxiety surrounding them while entering nursing homes.

Nursing home demographics reflect racial disparities in the provision of health care. It is widely recognized that a patient's race and gender might influence medical treatment and recommendations for care (Schulman, Berlin, Harless, Kerner, & Sistrunk, 1999). African Americans are four times more likely than their white counterparts to reside in substandard nursing homes (Mor, Zinn, Angelelli, Teno, & Millet, 2004). They are less likely to receive a range of medical options when they become ill (Chen, Rathore, Radford, Wang, & Krumholz, 2001) and are more likely to receive Medicaid to fund nursing home care.

There is documented disparity in treatment and access to health care (Berkman & Harootyan, 2003; Min, 2005; Tripp-Reimer, 1999). The more dependent a person is on Medicaid for nursing home payment, the more likely he or she is to receive poorer care (Farley & Allen, 1987; Mor et al., 2004). Economic disparities resulting in dependence on Medicaid funding and the greater likelihood of being placed in a lower-tier facility often mean less quality care. Lower-tier facilities are characterized by inadequate staffing levels, frequent changes in ownership, financial mismanagement, and are more likely cited for health-related deficiencies (Mor et al., 2004).

In "lower-tier" nursing homes, for example, where African Americans frequently reside, there are continual struggles with the provision of supportive care—too few wheel chairs, difficulty accessing products for incontinent patients, missing walkers, and a host of other conditions that actually work against the care of the older persons. Insufficient staffing and access to medical personnel makes the experience in the nursing home inadequate to support good health care for the resident. This is often a concern for families. There is a history characterized by medical mistreatment and health care exploitation, which results in distrust of the health care system and anxiety and fear when interacting with its services (Randall, 1996).

The rates of dementia and Alzheimer's disease among African Americans are higher than those among whites. Research suggests that the number of African Americans at risk for dementia will increase by more than 200 percent by 2030 (Borson & Katon, 1995; Gurland, Wilder, & Coleton, 1997). Even as the need for caregivers is increasing, generational or cohort changes within families may signal less of an availability or commitment to provide extensive in-home care. Long-term care facilities must be prepared to meet the needs of a growing population of African-American elders with dementia and debilitating illness that would require dedicated caregiving.

FAMILIES AND LONG-TERM CARE

The tradition of family caregiving within the African-American family has been impacted by changing generations, extended longevity, and availability of services. As the African-American family becomes more comfortable with the use of institutional social welfare systems, the reliance on informal family-based systems is reduced. Bowles study of African-American frail elders suggests that one could not assume generally that the elders receive family and church support (Bowles et al., 2000). The need for formal support is increasing.

When elders are placed in long-term care facilities, it is often a tumultuous time for caregivers. The concern regarding deteriorating health, quality of care, staff attentiveness, visitation, and financial matters are the issues that come to the forefront. The cultural responsiveness of the facility and the sensitivity of social workers and staff to cultural lifeways are very important. Family members sometimes set up a visitation system that is usually centered on the primary care-giver—the person who had been providing care prior to placement. The network may also include other immediate family, extended family, fictive kin, and the church members.

In health care facilities, residents and their family members may demonstrate displeasure with the treatment of medical staff, often suggesting certain folkways as more effective. This belief may persist even if it is not true and may be reflected in compliance difficulties within the nursing home setting. This may also reflect a history of distrust of the system as well as actual concern regarding treatment. The foundation of this intergenerational perspective may have been transmitted across multiple generations.

When the family members have experienced some form of inter-generational conflict, it is sometimes manifested through lack of visitation and responsiveness to the needs of the elderly resident in the nursing home. In these cases, there may be a need for staff to provide assistance to residents who rarely have visits from their families. Long-standing conflicts that sometimes exist over multiple generations may find their way into the caregiving experience and may need to be resolved, even after many years.

Mental health treatment is often not valued within the African-American elderly community. The stigma associated with such treatment is often linked to historical patterns of suspicion or religious teaching about mental illness. Often elders and their caregivers will not report or minimize symptoms. One of the common mental health disorders found among older adults, which is often underreported, is depression (Harralson, Tracela, Regenberg, & Micheal, 2002; Thomas & Sillin, 1972). Failure to diagnose depression in African-American elderly residents along with other disorders is often linked to stereotypical thinking (Williams, 1986) regarding the "happy-go-lucky" nature of older adults. This kind of thinking has led to misdiagnosis and suffering of residents who could have been benefited from receiving proper medication and treatment. The Teresik study (Teresik & Abrams, 2002) found that nurses tended to overrecognize depression, whereas social workers underrecognized depression among residents. These results clearly indicate the need for training in the identification and diagnosis of depression in African-American elders and sharing information. It is also important to recognize the strong connection between depression, disability, morbidity, and mortality (Harralson et al., 2002). It is not uncommon that long-term care residents suffer from a number of these conditions.

Care Receiving in African-American Families

Most older African Americans adhered to the belief that families were responsible to take care of their older adult family members—intergenerational caregiving. When a family is recognized as not providing care for a family member it is associated with shame.

During the early years of the twentieth century, institutional care was not sensitive to the needs of African Americans. In truth, both the private and the public systems failed to meet the needs of black families (Axinn & Levin, 1997). Exchanges with institutional systems were marked by mistreatment, racism, the inability to get needs met, distrust of institutional systems, and extreme discomfort. Office workers were often not polite to African Americans who were seeking services. African Americans were often served in substandard segregated spaces with little regard for personal privacy. Long-term care facilities are perceived as simply another institution and African-American residents often dread placement in a nursing home. Many negative messages about these facilities have been passed across generations.

A lack of reliance on these systems and distrust of them has become an intrinsic part of the perspective of many older African Americans.

As a result, elders in long-term care facilities most likely adopted the following coping styles:

1. *Reticence to speak:* Residents speak when spoken to and remain quiet otherwise.
2. *Reluctance to ask questions:* Even if they did not understand, they rarely asked questions.
3. *Compliance:* In a perceived hostile environment, they comply with those in authority under all conditions.
4. *Avoidance:* Avoid contact with social services or mental health providers.

The early life experiences that provided the catalysts for these behaviors may continue to impact daily interactions. Often younger family members must be diligent and serve as cultural interpreters or advocates for elder family members whose background and experience may significantly impact daily interactions.

Daily Life in Long-Term Care:
An Intergenerational Focus

Life in long-term care facilities presents a series of intergenerational relationships and caregiving opportunities. Often the staff are of different generations and sometimes of different races/ethnicities and cultural backgrounds. The need for cross-cultural understanding, sensitivity to residents' lifeways, and attention to generational cohort issues are paramount. These issues are particularly relevant as they relate to food preferences, personal care, communication, and interaction with other residents, staff, family, and extended family.

Food. Food is an important aspect of social life and is usually a centerpiece of meaningful social interactions. African-American elders' food preferences are linked to lifestyle, cultural lifeways, and economic status. It is not uncommon that African-American elders have strong preferences for fresh vegetables. Growing a garden was not only good exercise, but for poor people, it was a primary way to produce food in rural communities. Turnips, mustard and collard greens, kale, green beans, peas, and corn along with cornbread provided the core of a meal. Meat was often reserved for special occasions. Usually chicken was the most commonly eaten meat and only on special occasions. In the rural areas of the south, chicken, pigs, and cattle were raised and slaughtered for the family. Elderly residents will often place demands on family members to bring these kinds of dishes to the facility and if medically feasible and compatible with dietary restrictions, they should be allowed to do so.

Personal Care Issues. Respect is very important to African-American residents. The history of racism and discrimination in the United States reveals a deep and an abiding disrespect that was translated into behaviors that were discriminatory, racist, and designed to humiliate. As a result, respect based on the basic dignity and worth of the individual is critical to the African-American residents.

Bathing and personal care are private activities that often become less private in health care settings. Being touched or handled in private ways and having others see what has always been unseen except by the resident or close family is a violation of dignity. Although this kind of treatment may be necessary for the care of the resident, it is important for staff to find ways to demonstrate respect and to allow as much privacy as is possible.

Communication and Interaction. Language provides a picture of lifeways and experiences of African-American elders. Language reveals historical context, education, and mental status. Language is transmitted across generations; however, it is not uncommon that meaning is lost or distorted and leads to miscommunication. In addition, for African-American elder residents there may be certain terms that are expressed only in the presence of other African Americans or to family members.

Missy remembers:

> When I was a little girl people were not embalmed when they died. They were placed upon a cooling board and often remained at home for family visitation.

If Missy recounted this story, it would be important to ask, "What is a cooling board?" This is an example of language that has historical meaning, but if one did not live during the time period of Missy's birth, it would be critical to get clarification. Even the language used to describe African-American elders may need to be validated with the resident or relative. It would not be uncommon to call an older African American, "colored," black, African American, Negro, and so on. All of these terms are used appropriately at different times and in different contexts. When an elderly person uses a particular term to refer to African Americans that is not commonly used, a discussion must be held to determine common usage and meaning. Working with older African Americans might require learning some unfamiliar terms that are understood by the resident, but not known to the staff. Open communication is vital to understanding. Most importantly, listening provides important clues to understanding. Families can be a strong resource in helping to understand communication patterns and meaning. Facility staff should involve family to assist them in this matter.

Interaction with Other Residents. African-American elderly residents may be somewhat uncomfortable in social settings that involve interactions with whites or members of other ethnic groups. This discomfort may be temporary and may be based on limited opportunities to inter-act with whites in informal settings or interactions that were based on a system of inequality and injustice. Many older African Americans, seventy and older, lived in segregated communities and may have ste-reotypic thinking that they may feel uncomfortable with diverse groups of people. This often depends upon the life experiences of the individual. One might observe an African-American elder speaking to a white resident or a much younger staff person and referring to her as "Maam." This is not in deference to age but may be linked to per-ceived status differentials. Each resident has developed lifeways based on their lifetime experiences. Although these lifeways may not be rel-evant in all settings, there should be awareness that they exist.

Interaction Among Staff, Residents, and Relatives. Working with African-American residents and their families requires understanding some of the perceptions and distrust of social institutions, as previ-ously discussed. These attitudes and suspicions may impact interac-tions between staff, family members, and residents. It is critical for staff to demonstrate respect toward the resident and family members and an openness to allow inputs from the resident and family member/caregivers, in decisions regarding the resident. Some of these deci-sions may be complicated by different generational perspectives.

Unintentional prejudice, bias, and stereotypes may be demonstrated by staff toward African-American clients and their families. If this occurs, it may engender anger, resentment, and charges of discrimi-nation. Some families believe being vigilant is the only way to avoid these behaviors. When families are observed being hypervigilant, with regard to the resident, it is important to have a discussion in an open climate to facilitate sharing of concerns. Generalized fears that may have little actually to do with specific care issues in the nursing home may surface. Families must be allowed to share their concerns and fears and find mutual solutions. Discussion between the staff and family are critical, with a goal of increased understanding and reconciliation.

Recreational Activities. African-American elders often have differ-ent perspectives on recreation. Most have had a life with more work than leisure time. As a result, African-American elders may be unfa-miliar with some basic recreational activities found in long-term care facilities. Ping-pong, shuffleboard, and bridge may be activities not familiar to African-American elders. Black older adults often spend their leisure time in watching the "stories" (soap operas) or some males playing cards. Quilting, gardening, and knitting are activities that were vital to meeting family needs and are frequently considered recreational. Dancing and music may also be recreational activities found among African-American residents. Long-term care facility staff should be open to discussing recreational activities with residents and be flexible in their responses.

END-OF-LIFE CARE

African-American elders often utilize their spiritual beliefs to shape their perception of death and their preferences for end-of-life care (Wykle & Segal, 1991). Many African-American elders have little fear of death. They may have more fear about the circumstances of death rather than death itself. Being able to die a "good death," that is, free from suffering, long illness, and draining of financial resources of the family is a common desire. It is important to most African-American elders not to be a burden to the family in their end-of-life care.

The response to death depends on the age of death. African Americans tend to use the Bible as a standard for defining long life. Death at an old age, sometimes defined as seventy or older, is accepted as natural and normal. The place of death is also important. If given a preference, most African-American older adults would prefer to die at home with friends and family. It is not uncommon that final wishes involve being able to go home, even if the individual is in a long-term care facility.

African-American elders do not utilize hospice care to a significant degree. Only 8 percent of hospice patients are African Americans compared to 83 percent of white patients (Crawley, Payne, Bolden, Payne, & Washington, 2000). This underutilization of hospice care is owing to several factors. First, many are unaware that hospice care is available to them. Physicians must make referrals for hospice care, and lack of awareness often results in patients not taking advantage of this resource. Second, hospice care represents the involvement of another system outside of the family during the end of life, and African-Americans elders prefer to be cared for by family caregivers.

African Americans prefer life-prolonging measures in the treatment of terminal illnesses when compared to whites (Hopp & Duffy, 2000). This pattern may be representative of a distrust of institutional systems. There is a lingering concern that if given the opportunity, those in the dominant society would take advantage of African American and minorities and, poor care is motivated in part by racism and discrimination (Dilworth-Anderson et al., 2002). A number of studies have indicated that African Americans and the poor are often denied treatment options (Caralis, Davis, Wright, & Marcia, 1993; Randall, 1996). Denial of critical medical treatment is a fear of many African-American elders, and elders often believe that doctors have ultimate control over medical treatment. There is little awareness of patients' rights. Often the elder person may believe that medical staff are withholding certain medical information in an effort to protect or shelter (Caralis et al., 1993).

African Americans are less likely to complete living wills and other forms of advanced directives, such as do not resuscitate (DNR) orders (Hopp & Duffy, 2000). African Americans differ from European Americans both in their unwillingness to complete advance directives and their attitudes about life-sustaining treatment (Garrett, 1993). A study by Blackhall and colleagues (1995) found that when faced with a diagnosis of terminal illness, African-American elderly favored a patient autonomy-centered model of decision making rather than a family-centered model. The patient autonomy model suggests that African-American elders seek to make decisions about their own care, although they may heavily consider family wishes in this process. This result suggests that medical staff should ask a patient whether they want to involve their families in decision making about their care or whether they prefer the family to be provided with the information. Assumptions about family involvement may lead to inappropriate consideration of the patient's decision-making process.

African-American elders are not supportive of euthanasia or assisted suicide. Death is viewed as a transition often preceded by pain and suffering. The common belief is that if one can endure the suffering there will be relief through death at the proper time. This is an integration of traditional spiritual beliefs.

Many African-American elders believe in end-of-life planning. Funerals are an important statement about worth and value. It is also important to leave an inheritance to family members. Although this planning is not unusual, it is often done in an informal manner with families. Instructions may be written in the family Bible and usually one or more family members are informed about the wishes of the elder person.

IMPLICATIONS FOR SOCIAL WORK PRACTICE

Social work services must reflect an understanding of clients we serve. Without an accurate understanding of those whom we serve, intervention will not be appropriate. This chapter seeks to discuss caregiving and the historical context, lifeways as represented through traditions, rituals, behaviors, and customs that are a vital part of understanding the life stories of African-American elder clients and family caregiving.

The preference for family caregiving must be viewed as strength. Social workers can support family caregiving activities by providing information about formal supports that can be put in place to maintain elders in the home, coresidence living arrangement, or other noninstitutional placements. Intergenerational relationships also can be supported by facilitating good communication across generations, sharing information that assist the elder and the caregivers(s), and offering services when needed or requested.

Caregiving of African-American elders often reflects the utilization of coping strategies that may not be highly regarded within formal organizations. Reliance upon folk medicine, faith, and prayer may be seen in a negative light, although, there are a number of research studies suggesting the positive role of faith. (Peterson, 1990). Our understanding of person and environment transactions occurring over time is vital to developing interventions considering the many factors that shape the life course of every client. African-Americans elders and their families represent a rich tradition of strength and resilience, and these assets can be harnessed to provide the highest quality of appropriate intervention and possible care.

An increasing reliance upon care outside of the family context has led nursing home care to become an increasing option for many African-American families. Social workers within health care facilities must be vigilant in helping the medical staff diagnose changing medical conditions and in providing quality care to African-American elders. The tolerance of African-American elders for symptoms that are often called "old age-related" and the neglect in identifying early pain or other symptoms may lead to conditions that are undiagnosed. Every effort should be made to develop an ongoing relationship with medical personnel. Nurse's aides may be the most accurate source of information in diagnosing depression in African-American elders. Listening and asking appropriate questions will provide information necessary to understand the resident's condition and provide correct treatment.

Respect is a central element of caregiving for African-American elders. One of the important ways to demonstrate respect while interacting or involving in any personal care procedures is to make sure that the resident is addressed using proper names. In addition, asking or informing the resident of the procedures that will be used is important. For example, one might say:

> Mrs. Brown, I am about to assist you with your bath. Would you like me to help you to get into the tub?

> Mrs. Brown, it is time for me to get you back to your room; are you comfortable?

Although the staff is going through routine procedures, asking and informing the resident makes him or her feel respected and introduces some element of control. Simple actions such as knocking on a door before entering and asking preferences of the resident are important. The issue of respect is important to African-American elders. African-American residents can learn to interact comfortably in long-term care settings, but it may take some extra time. Usually through the process of adaptation, interactions between African-American and white and other ethnic group residents will begin to be more natural and appropriate. Language, stereotypes, and attitudes from past experiences should be encouraged to change.

When older African Americans become residents of health and long-term care facilities, food becomes an important part of the maintenance of lifeways familiar to the individual. Although health conditions may preclude eating some foods, vegetables, for example, are usually acceptable for most diets. One of the strategies that can be useful to assist in providing foods that are more familiar to African Americans is to utilize the resources available on-site. If there are African-American staff working in the kitchen, they might be able to work with the dietitian to occasionally have food commonly eaten by many African-American elders. Other African-American staff such as nurses or nursing assistants may be able to share favorite recipes that are more familiar to African-American residents. These strategies are fairly simple, and they help to facilitate the adaptation of older African-American residents.

CONCLUSION

The history of the experience of African Americans in the United States has promoted the development of unique lifeways and perspectives in individuals and families. African-American elders and their families have experienced a history of discrimination, oppression, and mistreatment, yet, they reflect the resilience and ability to survive. This survival is largely owing to strong family and extended family networks, intergenerational relationships, and a caregiving tradition. Family members often respect the tradition of providing care to elder relatives. With increased longevity and access to long-term care facilities, families have become more willing to place relatives in long-term care facilities. Also, some elders may not have younger relatives who are able to provide care. Human services agencies, and health and long-term care organizations must develop effective strategies to serve the needs of these residents. Effective care of African-American elders in health and long-term care organizations must reflect understanding of and responsiveness to the history, contributions, and culture. It must also recognize the intergenerational nature of caregiving in the African-American community and the role that the family and extended family members play when an elder must reside in a long-term care facility.

African-American older adults today are a composite of their predecessors, developing unique and characteristic perspectives and patterns of behavior. The story of African-American elders is a mosaic of triumph and tragedy, risk and resilience, and most of all transition and empowerment. Intergenerational approaches are well suited to working effectively with this population. Because of the connections that tend to exist across generations and the lifeways that are transmitted, understanding African-American elders must be couched within the context of history, tradition, culture, and rituals.

REFERENCES

Adams, V. H., & Jackson, J. (2000). The contribution of hope to the quality of life among aging African Americans: 1980-1992. *International Journal of Aging and Human Development, 50*(4), 279-295.

Antonucci, A. C. (1991). Strengthening the family support system of older minority person. In *Minority elders: Longevity, economics and health, building a public policy base* (pp. 32-37). Washington, DC: Gerontological Society of America.

Axinn, J., & Levin, H. (1997). *Social welfare: A history of the American response to need.* New York: Longman.

Baer, R. D., & Merrill, S. (1981). Toward a typology of black sectarianism as a response to racial stratification. *Anthropology Quarterly, 54,* 1-14.

Baer, R. D., & Nichols, J. (2001). Ethnic issues. In S. Loue and B. E. Quill (Eds.), *Handbook of Rural Health.* New York: Springer.

Bengtson, V. L., & Roberts, R. L. (1991). Intergenerational solidarity in aging families: An example of formal theory construction. *Journal of Marriage and the Family, 53*(4), 856-870.

Berkman, B., & Harootyan, L. (2003). *Social work and health care in an aging society.* New York: Springer.

Berrick, J. D. (1998). When children cannot remain home: Foster family care and kinship care. *The Future of Children, 8*(1), 72-87.

Blackhall, L. J., Murphy, G., Murphy, S., Frank, G., Michael, V., & Azen, S. (1995). *Ethnicity and attitudes toward patient autonomy.* Los Angeles: Department of Medicine, Pacific Center for Health Policy and Ethics, University of Southern California.

Bonner, G., Gorelick, P. B., Prohaska, T., Freels, S., Theis, S., & Davis, L. (1999). African American caregivers' preference for life-sustaining treatment. *Journal of Ethics, Law, and Aging, 5*(1), 3-15.

Borson, W., & Katon, W. (1995). Differential clinical characteristics of older black and white nursing home residents. *American Journal of Geriatric Psychiatry, 3,* 229-238.

Bowlby, J. (1988). A secure base: Clinical applications of attachment theory. London: Tavistock/Routledge.

Bowles, J., Brooks, T., Hayes-Reams, B., Butts, P., Myers, T., Allen, H., & Kingston, W. (2000). Frailty, family and church support among urban African American elderly. *Journal of Health Care for the Poor and Underserved, 11*(1), 87-99.

Cagney, K. A., & Agree, E. M. (1999). Racial difference in skilled nursing care and home health use: The mediating effects of family structure and social class. *Journal of Gerontology: Social Sciences, 54B,* S223-S236.

Callahan, J. (1996). Care in the home and other community settings: Present and future. In R. H. Binstock, L. E. Cluff, & Otto von Mering (Eds.), *The future of long-term care: Social and policy issues* (p. 320). Baltimore, MD: Johns Hopkins University Press.

Caralis, P., Davis, B., Wright, I., & Marcia, E. (1993). The influence of ethnicity and race on attitudes toward advance directives, life prolonging treatments and euthanasia. *Journal of Clinical Ethics, 4,* 155-165.

Carlton-LaNey, I. (2006). Rural African American caregiving. In B. Berkman (Ed.), *Handbook of Social Work in Health and Aging* (pp. 381-389). New York: Oxford University Press.

Chen, J., Rathore, S. S., Radford, M. J., Wang, Y., & Krumholz, H. M. (2001). Racial differences in the use of cardiac catheterization after acute myocardial infarction. *New England Journal of Medicine, 344,* 1443-1449.

Clarke, E. J., Preston, M., Raksin, J., & Bengtson, V. L. (1999). Types and conflicts and tensions between older parents and adult children. *The Gerontologist, 32*(6), 261-270.

Courtney, M. D., & Needell, B. (1997). Kinship foster care in Illinois. In J. D. Berric, R. Barth, & N. Gilbert (Eds.), *Child welfare research review: Vol. 2* (pp.130-149) New York: Columbia University Press.

Crawley, I., Payne, R., Bolden, J., Payne, T., & Washington, P. (2000). The initiative to improve palliative and end of life care in the African American community: Palliative and end of life care in the African American community. *Journal of the American Medical Association, 284,* 2518-2521.

Dilworth-Anderson, P., Williams, I. C., & Gibson, B. (2002). Issues of race, ethnicity and culture in caregiving research: A twenty year review (1980-2000). *Gerontologist, 42,* 237-272.

Ehrle, J., & Geen, R. (2002). Kin and nonkin foster care-findings from a national survey. *Children and Youth Services Review, 24,* 15-34.

Farley, R., & Allen. W. (1987). *The color line and the quality of life in America.* New York: Russell Sage Foundation.

Fuller-Thomson, E., & Minkler, M. (2000). American's grandparents caregivers: Who are they? In B. Hayslip Jr. and R. Goldberg-Glen (Eds.), *Grandparents raising grandchildren: Theoretical, empirical clinical perspectives* (pp. 3-21). New York: Springer Publishing Company.

Garrett, J. M. (1993). Life sustaining treatments during terminal illness: Who wants what? *Journal of General Internal Medicine, 8,* 361, 363.

Godkin, M. A., Wolf, R. S., & Pillemer, K. A. (1989). A case comparison analysis of elder abuse and neglect. *International Journal of Aging and Human Development, 28,* 207-225.

Gurland, B., Wilder, D., & Coleton, M. I. (1997). Differences in rates of dementia between ethno-racial groups. In L. G. Martin & B. Soldo (Eds.), *Racial and ethnic difference in the health of older Americans* (pp. 233-269). Washington, DC: National Academy Press.

Harralson, R., Tracela, M., Regenberg, A., & Micheal, B. A. (2002). Similarities and differences in depression among black and white nursing home residents. *American Journal of Geriatric Psychiatry, 10,* 175-184.

Hopp, F. P., & Duffy, S. (2000). Racial variations in end of life care. *Journal of the American Geriatric Society, 49,* 658-663.

Hummert, M. L., & Morgan, M. (2001). *Negotiating decisions in the aging family.* Mahwah, NJ: Lawrence Erlbaum and Associates.

Ingersoll-Dayton, B., Neal, M. B., Hammer, L. B. (2001). Aging parents helping adult children: The experience of the sandwiched generation. *Family Relations, 50*(3), 262-271.

Kopera-Frye, K., & Wiscott, R. (2000). Intergenerational continuity: Transmission. In B. Hayslip Jr. & R. Goldberg-Glen (Eds.), *Grandparents raising grandchildren: Theoretical empirical, clinical perspectives* (pp. 65-84). New York: Springer Publishing Company.

Mavundla, T. R. (1996). Factors leading to black elderly persons' decisions to seek institutional care in a home in the Eastern Cape. *Curationis, 19*(3), 47-50.

Min, J. W. (2005). Cultural competency: A key to effective future social work with racially and ethnically diverse elders. *Families in Society: The Journal of Contemporary Social Services, 86*(3), 347-358.

Minkler, M., Roe, K. M., & Price, M. (1992). The physical and emotional health of grandmothers raising grandchildren in the crack cocaine epidemic. *Gerontologist, 32,* 752-760.

Moody, H. R. (1996). Why dignity in old age matters. *Journal of Gerontological Social Work, 29,* 13-38.

Mor, V., Zinn, J., Angelelli, J., Teno, J. M., & Millet, S. C. (2004). Driven to tiers: Socioeconomic and racial disparities in the quality of nursing home care. *The Milbank Quarterly, 82*(2), 8202-8210.

Mutran, E. (1985). Intergenerational family support among blacks and whites: Response to culture or to socioeonomic differences. *Journal of Gerontology, 40,* 383-389.

National Alliance for Caregiving and AARP. (April, 2004). Caregiving in the U.S. Available online: www.metlife.com

National Center for Health Statistics. (2002). *Health disparities.* Available online: www.cdc.gov

O'Brien, P., Massat, C. R., & Gleeson, J. P. (2001). Upping the ante: Relative caregivers' perceptions of changes in child welfare policies. *Child Welfare, 80,* 719-748.

Peterson, J. (1990). Age of wisdom: Elderly black women in family and church. In J. Sokolovsky (Ed.), *The cultural context of aging* (pp. 213-228). New York: Bergin and Garvey Publishers.

Pinquart, M., & Sorensen, S. (2005). Ethnic differences in stressors, resources, and psychological outcomes of family caregiving: A meta-analysis. *Gerontologist, 45*(1), 90-106.

Randall, V. R. (1996). Slavery, segregation and racism: Trusting the health care system ain't always easy! An African American perspective on bioethics. *St. Louis University Publications Law Review, 15,* 191-235.

Schulman, K. A., Berlin, J. A., Harless, W., Kerner, J. F., & Sistrunk, S. (1999). The effect of race and sex on physicians' recommendations for cardiac catheterization. *The New England Journal of Medicine, 340*(8), 618-625.

Schulz, R., & Beach, R. S. (1999). Caregiving as a risk factor for mortality the caregiver health effects study. *JAMA, 282,* 2215-2219.

Spector, R. E. (2000). *Cultural diversity in health and illness.* Upper Saddle River, NJ: Prentice Hall.

Strom, R., Collingsworth, P., Strom, S., & Griswold, D. (1993). Strengths and needs of black grandparents. *International Journal of Aging and Human Development, 36,* 255-268.

Taylor, R. (1985). The extended family as a source of support to elderly blacks. *The Gerontologist, 25*(5), 488-495.

Taylor, R. J., Chatters, L. M., & Jackson, J. S. (1997). Introduction. In R. J. Taylor, J. S. Jackson, & L. M. Chatters (Eds.), *Family life in black America* (pp. 1-13). Thousand Oaks, CA: Sage.

Thomas, A., & Sillin, S. (1972). *Racism and Psychiatry.* New York: Brunner-Mazel.

Tripp-Reimer, T. (1999). Culturally competent care. In M. L. Wykle & A. B. Ford (Eds.), *Serving minority elders in the 21st century* (pp. 235-247). New York: Springer Publishing Company.

Williams, D. H. (1986). The epidemiology of mental illness in Afro-Americans. *Hospital and Community Psychiatry, 37*(1), 42-49.

www.marketsearch.com

Wykle, M., & Segal, M. (1991). A comparison of black and white family caregivers' experience with dementia. *Journal of the National Black Nurses Association, 5,* 29-41.

Chapter 10

Intergenerational Community Organizing

Jocelyn DeVance Taliaferro

If you want to have change, of course, the bottom line is that the folk for whom the change is meant must be involved in it.

Dorothy Cotton, civil rights activist

Healthy neighborhoods and communities are essential for healthy individuals and families to thrive. One mechanism for promoting healthy neighborhoods and communities is intergenerational community organizing and social action. Individuals of all ages have a role in the process of strengthening their neighborhoods and communities. This chapter discusses the opportunities and mechanisms, which are available and needed, for engaging multiple generations of African Americans in the community organizing process. It further highlights a discussion on the basic tenets of community organizing, the Afrocentric worldview, and intergenerational programming, and presents a model for intergenerational community organizing with African-American communities.

Community organizing is the process of mobilizing community members and providing the necessary resources for them to improve their own circumstances. It is a means of challenging the status quo, attempting to equalize social inequalities, and rebuking hegemonic, oppressive power systems (Schragge & Fisher, 2001). The purpose of community organizing is to promote social justice through transforming governance to be more pluralistic, policies to be more culturally relevant, and communities to be sources of support and development.

Social Work Practice with African-American Families

THE NEED

Community organizing is a tremendous tool for social justice and redistributive action. Within the context of social work profession, social action with the African-American community is essential. Intergenerational community organizing in these communities is particularly important owing to rising concerns of brain drain, an aging America, individualism, and the neoconservative agenda's assault on civil rights.

Brain Drain

As the African-American middle class shrinks, many opportunities for African-American youths and older adults disappear. The exodus of middle-class African Americans from traditionally minority communities leaves these communities vulnerable to the vagaries of external systems such as local political systems and real estate markets. Young people, and older adults, often leave these communities in search of better quality of life, superior school systems, higher paying jobs, and safer environments (Bankhead & Erlich, 2005; Domina, 2006). This brain drain, where the best and brightest of the community leave, has a damaging effect and leaves these communities and neighborhoods on the periphery of prosperity.

Aging of the Population

At the turn of the century, life expectancy was only forty-six years. Today, life expectancy is approximately seventy-six years. By 2030, the number of Americans over eighty-five will double and by 2050, 40 percent of the population will be older than fifty (Miles, 1999). At that time, older adults will outnumber children and youths. Many pundits have predicted that the aging of America will create a huge burden on the society as it has to face a majority of members who traditionally require care and are heavily dependent on others. However, this is not necessarily so. The feeble, fragile, older adult has given way to the active and activist individual. Older adults are taking a much more efficacious stance regarding their aging process and needs. Rather than having decisions made for them, older adults are bringing their activist roots with them and influencing government agencies, health care organizations, and financial institutions. Armed with knowledge and skill they are questioning the prevailing hegemony, processes, and policies; making decisions; enriching their lives; and demanding attention.

Increased Individualism

In the United States, the dominant culture ideology professes that individual effort and personal motivation leads to success. Moreover, if an individual is not successful, it is believed to be a result of personal weakness rather than any societal influence. This individual responsibility ideology promotes a "blame the victim" mentality, condemns the individual as a failure, and excuses society from the responsibility of providing assistance to the less fortunate (Katz, 1989). The belief that poor people are responsible for their own plight is used to validate the current system of governance and social policies. In this tradition, Americans value individual and property rights above social justice and redistribution (Gilens, 1999). Therefore, community organizing must continue to foster an ideology of a healthy interconnectedness of individuals in communities. Although African-American communities have historically rejected this ideology, owing to a rise in neoconservativism, there has been a shift toward this paradigm.

Neoconservatism and the Decline of Civil and Human Rights

The neoconservative movement, which has been promoted by the political systems of the twenty-first century, poses a challenge to human and civil rights (Bankhead & Erlich, 2005). The Bush administration's Uniting and Strengthening America by Providing Appropriate Tools Required to Intercept and Obstruct Terrorism (USA PATRIOT Act) Act of 2001 and National Security Agency's classified domestic surveillance program (domestic spying program) have begun to incrementally dismantle the human and civil rights of American citizens. Although racial profiling of African Americans may have been replaced (to some degree) by individual profiling from the Middle East, these and other intrusive practices have become more acceptable in terms of protection from terrorism. Therefore, it is essential that rights campaigns and community organizing continue to emerge from American communities.

On the basis of continued need for community organizing, there is an opportunity for the development of a set of tenets for these activities within the African-American community. Before the discussion of such a model, it is important to discuss the basic assumptions and models of community organizing.

COMMUNITY ORGANIZING

Community organizing seeks to restructure institutions and rearrange power structures to bring widespread social change. It was born out of protests against inequality, powerlessness, and overbearing government control can be found in the efforts to gain civil rights and end discrimination (Gittell & Vidal, 1998; Schragge & Fisher, 2001). Within this spirit of conflict, the historic foundation of community organizing is the strengthening of relationships among people and organizations sharing similar values and interests (Stoecker, 2003).

Community organizing is not only a set of techniques but also a way of viewing the world, a paradigm using justice, social responsibility, self-determination, and change as parameters. Community organizing has a multitude of meanings, and for the purpose of this discussion the following definition is taken into consideration: "Community organizing is not just a means to win issues, but also to build powerful community organizations, in the process of which community relationships are rebuilt and individuals are empowered" (Stoecker, 2003, p. 494).

Theoretical Underpinnings of Community Organizing

Community organizing is characterized by several basic tenets. The interchange of concepts such as community, power, empowerment, and leadership are essential components of any community organizing campaign.

Community

Communities have traditionally been considered as spaces where residents, in close proximity, shared goods, resources, and services are separated from other geographic areas (Christenson, Fendley, & Robinson, 1989). These areas are sources of support and connection

(Peterman, 2000). Owing to the mobility of today's society, communities are becoming more difficult to identify. Generally there are two types of communities—identificational and traditional (Kirst-Ashman & Hull, 2006; Schriver, 2004). Identificational communities are those that primarily focus on common interest. Individuals in identificational communities may be bound by geography or location, but what is of greater importance are the shared interests and ways of living (i.e., the social work or legal community).

However, the primary focus of this chapter is on traditional communities, where individuals are connected by geography and location. Communities are characterized by "residences, shared living space, and some array of businesses that serve the needs of those who live there" (Kirst-Ashman & Hull, 2006, p. 253). Communities provide the arena for social interaction, group identity, security, and resources, including education, health, housing, and cultural sustenance (Ewalt, Freeman, & Poole, 1998).

Power and Empowerment

Generally, community organizing campaigns emerge from a need to redistribute power relationships. In its most simple form, power is exhibited when one person's will takes precedence over all other intentions or interests (Biklen, 1983). Power within the context of community organizing means that people who are disenfranchised and marginalized are provided with the freedom to think, decide, and govern themselves based on what is in their own best interests.

Within the community organizing context, the power of state and local polity directly influences the viability of community organizing efforts. Those who have power seldom want to relinquish it, making community organizing necessary, especially for nondominant populations. In a system where decision-making bodies, both formal and informal, serve to benefit those who already have resources and influence, there is little room for redistribution of power, creating the necessity for community organizing efforts.

Beyond power, empowerment is central to community organizing. Empowerment is the self-determination of residents to identify their own problems and address them as they deem reasonable (Chekki, 1979; Mondros & Wilson, 1994). An empowered community is able to manage itself because of sustained involvement and control of service delivery and governing structures. To obtain this goal, the use of democratic structures is needed to ensure that service users or community representatives have a voice and ultimately control (Alinsky, 1946). This internal problem-solving method is opposed to externally imposed forces, structures, or ideologies.

Empowerment relies on democratic participation, also a major theme in community organizing, which provides a vehicle for ordinary citizens, especially from nondominant groups, to engage and participate in local governance and decision making. It is a way of raising voice to those who often cannot be heard over the din of the elite dominant members of the polity (Biklen, 1983; Schragge & Fisher, 2001). Community organizing promotes genuine democratic processes to accomplish the empowerment goals of community organizing through citizen participation (Chekki, 1979).

Empowerment increases the esteem of community members by increasing human capital and capacity, which adds to the momentum of community organizing efforts (Chaskin, Joseph, & Chipenda-Dansokho, 1998; Kahn, 1992). As individuals gain success in their small efforts, and issues get resolved, personal power, self-efficacy, and self-determination are enhanced for those who participate and win, thereby illuminating the power of supporting one another and working cooperatively (Kahn, 1992).

Leadership

Leadership is essential to community organizing, because the strength of personal relationships helps to drive the organizing process. Within the context of community organizing, leadership involves either hiring an outside professional organizer to mobilize residents, or recruiting leaders among the members of the community. The goal of using residents is to cultivate and build on the existing competencies of community residents (Delgado, 1994; Eichler, 1995; Gittell & Vidal, 1998). Most often, individuals are mobilized by local, native leadership— possibly with the guidance of a professional organizer. The leader helps the community frame the issues, whereas the community members choose the issues to pursue (Mondros & Wilson, 1995) Many community residents, both older adults and youths, gain valuable political and social capital while serving in these roles (Warren, 2001).

HISTORICAL TRADITIONS OF COMMUNITY ORGANIZING IN THE AFRICAN-AMERICAN COMMUNITY

Community organizing has a long history in the redistributive and social justice activities of African-American communities. Multiple strategies are used by community members as they create space to accommodate change and social justice (Guitierrez, Alvarez, Nemon, & Lewis, 1996). Within community organizing, three dominant models have emerged and are currently utilized by practitioners. These models include *consensus organizing, conflict-based,* and *institution-based community organizing.* The discussion that follows examines the unique goals, strategies, and structures of these approaches, and how they have manifested in the African-American experience.

Consensus Organizing

Consensus organizing is a method of social change that emphasizes collaboration and partnership building. According to the Consensus Organizing Institute (Eichler, 1995), the guiding principles of consensus organizing include indigenous leadership, empowerment, the ability to harness and make compatible multiple self-interests, and sustainability of relationships. Consensus organizing seeks to include all stakeholders, which often transcends traditional community barriers or boundaries. The goal of the strategy is to build new institutions and collaborations rather than work within existing structures. The creation of a new entity is thought to lessen the effects of turf wars and self-interest, thereby leveling the playing field for all participants. Consensus organizing posits that confrontation is not always as effective a method as collaboration (Eichler, 1995). Consensus organizing revises conceptualizations of power in that power is not a zero-sum arrangement but a malleable and distributable article. Often the participants make strange bedfellows, but consensus organizing does not eliminate anyone as a potential partner or collaborator.

The foci of this type of organizing are the common interests, rather than the uneven power relationships or control of social institutions. The method of decision making is that of participatory democracy. It is important to note that consensus organizing does have a darker side, explicitly its conceptualizations of power (Stoecker, 2003) and the historical vulnerability of minorities, women, and low-income individuals in negotiation processes (Northouse, 2003).

However, consensus organizing focuses on capacity building through the creation of linkages to larger entities, such as public and private, government, and nonprofit agencies. It is anticipated that these linkages will enhance relations, which will provide access and control over the agenda for the community (Eichler, 1995; Gittell & Vidal, 1998).

Most notably, during the Progressive Era, responses to institutional racism and oppression forged the development of several organizations, including the National Association of Colored women, the Committee on Urban Conditions Among Negroes (currently the National Urban League), and the National Association for the Advancement of Colored People (NAACP). These organizations often developed out of the consensus organizing tradition due to the lack of power within the African-American community. The need to include "others" and individuals outside the community to gain power was the basis for many of these organizational arrangements and partnerships.

Well beyond the Progressive Era, inequality (including racism, sexism, and sexual exploitation) and poverty (and its attendant issues such as civil rights, unemployment, hunger, homelessness, substandard housing, and education) continued to be the hallmark issues of community organizing in African-American communities. Fighting these multiple "-isms" have been "Inextricably connected to race uplift" (Carlton-LaNey, 2001, p. xiii). In addition to the intense African-American social action of the Progressive Era, the 1960s reflected the strong traditions of African-American social justice and civil rights activism, particularly in the conflict-based organizing model.

Conflict-Based Community Organizing

The power base of traditional community organizing rests in the potential consolidation of individual voices of community members. Where powerful people have organized resources, direct community organizing relies on mobilized people. Conflict-based organizing is flexible in structure, but is militant as it is flexible. The strategies used for these campaigns include protests, media attention campaigns, sit-ins, and other contestation methods. The disadvantage of the direct membership organizing is that group members are often filled with righteous indignation regarding their issue but have little more than that in the way of resources. Within the context of present day community organizing, these campaigns are often short lived and have cohesion difficulties when transitioning to the next issue (Warren, 2001).

The dominant culture attributes the development of this form of organizing to Saul Alinsky and his Chicago-based Back of the Yards community action in the 1950s; however, this type of direct conflict can be seen in the slave experiences of Denmark Vesey in Charleston, South Carolina in 1822 and Nat Turner at Southampton County, Virginia, in 1831. Icons such as Ida B. Wells, Marcus Garvey, and Malcolm X all held "political ideologies in direct opposition to the power elite" (Carlton-LaNey, 2001, p. xiv). These organizers used conflict organizing strategies and worked with existing African-American community institutions or created new ones to build relationships and develop bonding social capital (e.g., the lateral relationships among community members based on trust and reciprocal relationships). The bonding social capital was ultimately transformed into political and bridging social capital (e.g., the relationships external to the community that garners resources to generate development and improvement) (Guitierrez et al., 1996). African-American community organizing builds on this tradition of organizing from the Civil Rights era (Guitierrez et al., 1996).

The tactics of African-American community organizing have ranged from direct with the development of the Organization of Afro-American Unity (OAAU) and Black Panthers to consensus as evidenced by the Congress for Racial Equality (CORE) and the NAACP. In addition to consensus and conflict organizing, institution-based organizing, was the linchpin of organizations such as the Congress for Racial Equality (CORE) and activities such as the Freedom Schools. From the activities of these organizations and others (see Day, 2003 and Trattner, 1999) African Americans initiated community organizing and social action campaigns across the country, some of the most well-known examples of institution-based community organizing being the Montgomery County bus boycott that began in 1955 and lasted for 381 days and the historic March in Washington in 1963.

Institution-Based Community Organizing

Institution-based organizing evolved as a variation to conflict-based organizing. The conflict-based, direct confrontation, with zero-sum outcomes, often does not meet the long-term needs of communities that have to sustain mobilization and participation efforts to accomplish community change and improvement. Institution-based organizing focuses on organizational membership, relational organizing, mixed strategies, and leadership capacity building. The hallmark of these institution-based organizing entities is that their membership is made up of *organizations* rather than *individuals.* The organizations that are recruited for membership are generally well-entrenched institutions (e.g., churches, unions) within the community (Warren, 2001). The member organizations already have a significant power base within the community that when collectively galvanized gives the resulting organization political leverage and allows the member organizations to be "players" on the political landscape (Delgado, 1997).

The strategies and tactics used by institution-based organizing are a hybrid of conflict and consensus methods. These mixed strategies include demonstrations as well as large-scale public meetings that increase accountability and pressure, for instance, holding government officials and others accountable to the community for any promises or commitments made during the campaign trail (Delgado, 1997). Contemporary examples of institution-based organizing include Southern Echo, which began in 1989 and transformed into an institution-based organization that works with and in support of African-American and working class community leadership and organizations throughout rural Mississippi and organizations in eleven other Southern states. Similarly Baltimoreans United in Leadership Development (BUILD) has a membership primarily of African-American religious congregations and is one of the largest predominantly African-American local community organizations in the country. For more than twenty years BUILD has launched successful living wage campaigns and championed community engagement. BUILD's activities reflect its affiliation with the Industrial Areas Foundation (IAF), a national network of community advocacy groups. Institution-based organizing promotes long-term involvement and relationship building among the member organizations to carry out these types of maintenance tasks.

The community organizing strategies, whether consensus, conflict, or institutional, have been effective in bringing the issues of racism, segregation, Jim Crowism into the mainstream consciousness. For example, the Black Panthers "protested rent evictions, informed welfare recipients of their legal rights, taught classes in African American history, and demanded school traffic lights in a street where several African American children had been killed while crossing" (Day, 2003, p. 322). These activities and other were indicative of the social action activities that were mounted throughout United States history. The proliferation of self-help organizations, including National Association of Colored Women, sororities, fraternities, and the aforementioned community organizations, speaks to the entrenchment of activism, organizing, and mobilization in the African-American community (Cook, 2001).

Therefore, based on the current needs of local communities and the historic tradition of African-American social activism, there is an opportunity to develop methods explicitly for working with multiple generations in the African-American community. The following is a discussion of a framework necessary for developing a model of African-American intergenerational community organizing.

AFRICAN-AMERICAN INTERGENERATIONAL COMMUNITY ORGANIZING AS A MODEL

Intergenerational community organizing with African Americans must be grounded in the (1) celebration of African-American culture, (2) bridging of the gap between generations, and (3) opportunities for leadership development. Figure 10.1 illustrates how each of the aspects of the effort must be layered. Community organizing in its traditional form can be coupled with intergenerational activities that are consistent with an Afrocentric perspective. Although community organizing tenets have already been discussed, the following discussion will reflect the methods of infusing intergenerational practice and an Afrocentric perspective into the community organizing process.

Intergenerational Community Organizing

As discussed in other chapters of this book, intergenerational programs provide opportunities for interaction, engagement, and reflection where both older adults and youths have an opportunity to reconsider

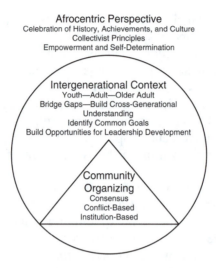

FIGURE 10.1. A Model of Intergenerational Community Organizing with African Americans

previously held notions (Kaplan & Liu, 2004). Guiding principles of intergenerational community organizing, therefore, should include "reciprocity, united to common purpose, reflection, partnerships, and preparation and support" (Scannell & Roberts, 1994, p. 8). These principles of intergenerational programming as discussed in other chapters, (see—Waites, Williams, Leach & Becker; Brodie & Gadling) provide the basic framework for general intergenerational programming.

Scannell and Roberts (1994) and Kaplan (1997) provide an overview of traditional components of intergenerational community serving and organizing projects. Specifically, participants have the opportunity to revisit their role as citizens and either to renew or gain a perspective on the importance of civic engagement. These activities foster active citizenry in their shared community. Residents are able to learn and participate in the legislative and community activist process (Ginwright, 2005; Kaplan, 1997). They are able to conceptualize new models of social change and understand that they can impact the political and policy-making process. Examples of intergenerational community organizing or community development programs include SETS, Hidden Treasure, Language Link, and Neighborhoods 2000 (for an extended discussion of these programs see Kaplan, 1997). These service-learning programs focus on a myriad of issues from cultural and historical preservation to human service provision.

Intergenerational community organizing activities have the potential to provide opportunities to engage community leaders, such as politicians, and make the political process relevant, tangible, and accessible to participants. These intergenerational partnerships often illuminate the fact that community goals of youths and older adults are often very similar (Kaplan, 1997). Both groups are concerned with issues of crime and safety, environment, and community beautification.

These programs sometimes make esoteric issues relevant by providing information from a personal perspective and presenting issues from a life span perspective. For instance, in intergenerational environmental programs, youths and older adults are able to see how the environment is important to youths as a necessary resource to be protected for their own use, and for older adults as a resource to be preserved for the use of their children and children's children.

Furthermore, youths begin to see the historical context of the current struggles and are able to recognize transitions and the cyclical nature of historical events. Youths are also introduced to the historical context of African-American struggles with racism, sexism, and classism. Both groups are able to provide each other with "stereotype-breaking experiences [that have] self-affirmation value—the value of being understood as you are, rather than how the media presents you" (Kaplan, 1997, p. 218).

In addition, although there is a substantial amount of literature about the benefits of intergenerational programming from the perspective of youths, fewer reports highlight the benefits to older adults, other than being service recipients (Scannell & Roberts, 1994). However, Kaplan and Liu (2004) suggest that older adults develop more positive views of young people; enjoy quality of life enhancements including better physical and mental health; feel useful in that they can share their life's wisdom and experiences; and, are able to serve as true elders and leaders in the community.

Moreover, intergenerational programming provides the foundation for teaching important values. In the case of intergenerational community organizing with African Americans, the value of activism can be instilled. Although many of intergenerational programs are not long enough to create full-fledged activists, it does provide the foundation for recognizing the need for the work of improving lives and changing communities. Exposure to the myriad of issues and the need for community and social action provides the training ground for the birth of an activist perspective among youths. It provides the structured and nurturing environment in which youths can try their proverbial wings with the promise of guidance and support.

Celebration of African-American Culture

In developing a model for African-American intergenerational community organizing, it is essential to explore the issues of race and culture as not to perpetuate a culture of oppression and inequality. Even looking at communities as though they were colorblind is detrimental, because it denies the impact of race and ethnicity, which in fact adds to the richness of communities of color. Colorblindness further denies the impact of oppression on the population by clinging to a myth of equal opportunity. Therefore, culture must be recognized and celebrated to avoid perpetuating the problems that community organizing is meant to ameliorate.

Those interested in community organizing with African Americans must acknowledge the strength and resilience of these communities. After dealing with centuries of oppression and injustice, African Americans have had to develop significant survival strategies and mechanisms of dealing with the vagaries of an unjust society. That historical and lived reality has required the development of many strengths that should be highlighted during the organizing process (Guitierrez et al., 1996).

One way to do that is to embrace an Afrocentric perspective or "African self-consciousness" (Schiele, 2000). Jerome Schiele (2000) asserts that the African self-consciousness "can be succinctly defined as a state of awareness among African Americans that they are a cultural group and that their behavior should be aimed at fostering the collective survival, advancement, and prosperity of people of African ancestry" (p. 19). As such, African-American community organizing must have an acknowledgement of, and appreciation for, the cultural, historical, and collective experience of African Americans. The Afrocentric perspective seeks to inform the consciousness of African

Americans so that they celebrate the achievements and culture of African Americans.

Within this context, the seven principles of the Nguzo Saba are instructive. The Nguzo Saba is traditionally connected with annual Kwanzaa celebration. Since its creation by Maulana Ron Karenga in 1966, Kwanzaa has been an annual celebration of community, family, and culture held between December 26 and January 1 (see Pleck, 2001). Since 1983, Kwanzaa has gained appeal and widespread acceptance, especially among middle-class African Americans (Pleck, 2001).

The principles of the Nguzo Saba are given in Table 10.1, which lists each principle in Swahili with its pronunciation and English

TABLE 10.1. Principles of the Nguzo Saba

Principle (Pronunciation)	Meaning	Description
Umoga (OO-MOE-JAH)	Unity	A commitment to the idea of togetherness in which healthy families build healthy communities, and without unity neither the family nor the community can survive.
Kujichagulia (CO-GEE-CHA-GOO-LEE-AH)	Self-determination	A commitment to take the responsibility for achievement upon ourselves as the essence of freedom.
Ujima (OO-GEE-MA)	Collective work and responsibility	Encourages self-criticism and personal evaluation as it relates to the common good of the family/community. Progress is impossible without collective work and struggle.
Ujamaa (OO-JAH-MAH)	Cooperative economics	Belief that wealth and resources should be shared. On the national level, cooperative economics can help African Americans take physical control of their own destinies.
Nia (NEE-AH)	Purpose	The belief in the necessity for each individual to examine his or her ability to put his or her skill or talent to use in the service of the family and community at large.

TABLE 10.1 *(continued)*

Principle (Pronunciation)	Meaning	Description
Kuumba (KOO-M-BAH)	Creativity	Building and developing our creative potential involves both aesthetic and material creations. It is essential that creativity be encouraged in all aspects of African-American culture. It is through new ideas that we achieve higher levels of living and a greater appreciation for life.
Imani (E-MAH-NE)	Faith	A belief in ourselves as individuals and as a people as well as the power of God that is greater than us.

Source: Adapted from Karenga, 2006; Pleck, 2001.

translation (Karenga, 2006). It also provides an explanation of the principle in relationship to African-American culture.

The principles of the Nguzo Saba, can be incorporated and explicitly highlighted during the community organizing process. The collectivist principles, specifically unity and collective work and responsibility, express the value of social responsibility, which can be the catalyst of the organizing effort (Guitierrez et al., 1996). Helping the participants in intergenerational community organizing to understand that the essence of social justice, making sure that no one is marginalized, is consistent with intergenerational community organizing with African Americans. The ideology of "I am because we are" provides a framework and foundation upon which to explain why the work of organizing is so very important. Infusing the collectivist consciousness that "I am my brother's keeper" is consistent with an Afrocentric worldview. This perspective is juxtaposed against an increasingly individualistic ideology of the United States. However, focusing African-American communities on the legacy and history of a collectivist worldview is tremendously helpful to developing the foundation for building traditional community organizing strategies.

In addition, the collectivist principle of the Nguzo Saba, empowerment, or self-determination, as discussed, is a cornerstone of community organizing. To be able to make decisions, govern, and find solutions to one's own problems is tremendously important in fostering other Nguzo Saba principles such as creativity and purpose for African Americans. As part of the Afrocentric perspective, the ability to cast off the images and portrayals that have been imposed by others is constitutive to self-awareness and the creation of an authentic self. The authentic self is one that operates within the understanding of a life purpose, one that is cooperative, and moves in harmony with others and God (Schiele, 2000).

Recognizing the contributions of all generations, participating in cultural ceremonies, learning African and African-American history, including the contributions to the history of community organizing, and taking on cultural humility (see Hunt, 2001) are all ways to celebrate African-American culture. Incorporating rites of passage activities, teaching and learning about African-American heros and heroines, and their contributions are fundamental to the framework of community organizing with African Americans.

Bridge the Gaps Between Generations

Intergenerational community organizing with African-American communities "creat[es] more shared public spaces that foster social connectedness, and provid[es] ongoing opportunities for open dialogue between diverse groups are all potential vehicles for promoting interdependence and a new kind of citizenship in communities" (Henkin & Kingson, 1998, p. 103). Intergenerational community organizing assists in framing the issue, problem, and solution within the history and cultural experience of people of color (Guitierrez et al., 1996), specifically African Americans. Adults provide the richness of context required for understanding the internal and external forces that affect the problem, the solutions, the actors, targets, and orientation and can provide the infrastructure for mobilizing community organizing campaigns and youth. While youths have ideas and energy, older adults have seen it, done it, and lived it (HoSang, 2003). Elders must encourage youths to bring their new perspectives to the old problems of racism, sexism, and classism; as the wise man Solomon said, there is nothing new under the sun. This combination targeted at promoting intergenerational solutions to community problems has the potential to be powerful and catalytic.

Given the strengths of each group, it is important for older adults to provide this environment without squelching the ideas, eagerness, and excitement of youths (Guitierrez et al., 1996). Although it may not have worked during the 1900s, 1950s, or even 1990s, it may work today due to changes in systems, regimes, context, and the culmination of small victories of the past. These circumstances may have, in fact, paved the way for success among current youth.

Because community organizing is most effective when several groups with divergent interests are coalesced around a particular issue, it is effective to see older adults and youths, who at face value may be in competition for resources, come together for a common goal (Guitierrez et al., 1996). This type of coalition building often breeds strange bedfellows for the purpose of goal attainment, thereby identifying collective goals and bringing together older adults and youths where their common interests intersect provides the basis for community organizing.

Within this milieu, it is important to avoid pitting old and young against one another. In the competitive nature of the United States context, systems are often inclined to reduce intergenerational interactions to competition over scarce resources (Henkin & Kingson, 1998). This paradigm should be rejected and debates should be reframed. In essence, the goal of intergenerational community organizing should be to focus on solutions to collective problems, eliminating the need for zero-sum arrangements. For example, the discourse regarding the solvency of Social Security has the potential to create conflicts between older and younger generations, particularly African-American youths. The fact that Social Security is the retirement plan for many African Americans and the idea that unprecedented numbers of older adults will use Social Security have tremendous potential to complicate intergenerational organizing around Social Security. However, there is an opportunity to look at the issue more holistically and address the real problem rather than place blame. Efforts taken to exploring why so many African Americans rely on Social Security as their sole source of retirement income, examining the effects of privatization on the African-American community, and developing strategies to address remaining cultural inequality is better than fighting about

Social Security insolvency. These delicate issues are the nexus of an intergenerational approach to addressing Social Security for African Americans.

Beyond issue-based conflicts, one of the more obvious tensions is the generational gaps in communication and expression (Ginwright, 2005). The hip-hop culture is extremely prevalent among American youths. Older adults may have a disdain or low tolerance for the different modes of expression prevalent in hip-hop culture, which comes with its own set of norms and mores. However, it is important that these differences be transcended in the community organizing process.

Hip-hop culture is characterized by the four elements of MCing, DJing, graffiti art, and break dancing (Alridge, 2005; Stovall, 2006). DJing, specifically sampling, and rap are excellent resources for making intergenerational connections. Sampling, (i.e., the infusion of sounds or voices, often from well-known social artifacts, into a song) provides a connection between the music and values of the two generations (Alridge, 2005). Many of the sounds that are sampled are from music and historical events that would be quite familiar to older adults. As an example, the music of James Brown, Stevie Wonder, and the Stylistics as well as the words from the speeches of Malcolm X and Martin Luther King Jr. are often heard in contemporary hip-hop music. Rap, specifically socially conscious rap, is an opportunity to connect the struggle of African-American youths to that of the Civil Rights era (see Alridge, 2005 for an extended discussion of the civil rights connection between hip-hop and civil rights).

Opportunities for Leadership Development and Mentoring

Beyond coalescing around issues and generational differences, a significant point of concern regarding intergenerational programming is the level of youths' involvement and shared power. Finding the appropriate balance in decision making and responsibility is often difficult. Many youths in urban areas have significant experience and much to share; therefore, if they are not given a voice in governance of the effort, they may resent not having decision-making authority (Ginwright, 2005). Many youths must deal with adult-like day-to-day life pressures (e.g., caregiving, employment, navigating human service systems) as well as the critical issues of the youths (e.g., identity development, belonging, sexuality) (HoSang, 2003). These personal problems, that are often a result of environmental tensions, affect the intergenerational relationship because of the psychological and physical impacts on the individual members (Ginwright, 2005).

Older adults have to be sensitive to these issues, often times before the community organizing activities begin. Under these circumstances, there is opportunity for change and development. Individuals are often open to change and trying new things during a crisis (Visser, 2004). Therefore, these life pressures and critical issues may present opportunities to engage youths in community organizing to ameliorate those basic needs and imminent threats. However, individuals are also often unable to work on higher level goals during a crisis because the personal crisis takes center stage and lessens the importance of other affairs (Visser, 2004).

Welfare reform and decreased wages have pushed many adolescents into the more adult roles of caretaker and provided them with decision-making power in the home environment (Ginwright, 2005). As youths engage in these adult-like behaviors, it changes traditional conceptualizations of the role of youths in intergenerational programming. Traditional understandings are that youths should have decision-making power and a voice in the activities, foci, and direction of intergenerational programming. However, some young people, because of their very much adult-like responsibilities relish the opportunity to give decision making over to their older adult partners. To some older adults it may appear that youths are passively engaged. However, it may be that they are simply happy to participate as a child, abdicating governance responsibilities to the adults (Ginwright, 2005). Negotiating this terrain is important to the cohesiveness of the community organizing partners and ultimately the success of any community organizing campaign.

In spite of these decision-making minefields, it is essential that youths be afforded leadership opportunities. Providing leadership development and mentoring opportunities within the intergenerational community that organizes with African-Americans' framework is essential. Older adults have a special role in this development process, to act as the "elders of the tribe." Older adults provide the perspective of generations by creating a sense of hope and not despair (Henkin & Kingson,

1998). Community organizing is often a long-term activity where strides or success are, most often, not immediately evident. When youths might feel discouraged, the resiliency of older adults under similar, and some may say harsher, conditions may serve as an inspiration for youths.

In contrast, these activities have the potential to ignite older adults' enthusiasm and stimulate new ideas and perspectives on old problems (HoSang, 2003). Many community organizing campaigns have been long-suffering (e.g., minimum wage, affordable housing, health care access) and the new insight of youths may be what is needed to rejuvenate some of these old campaigns. Adults can serve as "mentors, political strategists, trainers, and fundraisers" (HoSang, 2003, p. 68).

Mentoring is a common approach to meet the needs of African-American youths, and provides intergenerational arrangements and interactions. However, it is imperative that the reciprocal learning process continues throughout the community organizing activities so that older adults and youths get to experience as mentor and teacher. Activities such as experience sharing, skills development through role-plays, and brainstorming sessions provide opportunities for leadership development from a nonauthoritarian perspective.

Within the community organizing tradition, leadership cultivated from within the community is most often desired (see Alinsky, 1946; Guinier, 1994). Community youths should be encouraged to take on the leadership mantle and supported by older adults (Guitierrez et al., 1996). Older adults should consider operating from less direct roles than a leader, and instead serving as consultant or technical assistant. Many community scholars suggest that individuals who can create intimate interpersonal relationships among community members are the best leaders (Ganz, 2002; Guitierrez et al., 1996). Adults can help to make linkages and referrals, serving as a liaison to the community and larger systems and providing models of collaboration for youths to emulate.

In addition, regarding leadership, often youths have not yet been introduced to traditional systems and are not at high risk of co-optation. Therefore, youths can serve as community leaders without fear of retribution. They often do not have the constraints of political requirements to stifle their ability to speak freely. However, they need to recognize that others may have such limitations. The community residents with "good government jobs" or other assets at risk may be less likely to challenge existing governance systems outwardly for fear of reprisal.

Challenges to the Model

Like the critiques of traditional community organizing, the preliminary model of community organizing with African Americans has its challenges. It is important to remember that "the African-American community" is not monolithic and does not lend itself to singular strategies to address the myriad perspectives and concerns of its communities. However, the proposed model is one way of using traditional community organizing concepts and theories within the context of intergenerational community organizing with African Americans.

Although intergenerational programming will not solve all problems of the United States, it is one option for strengthening the social compact of the nation (Henkin & Kingson, 1998). The goal is to focus on needs of multiple generations and celebrate everyone's contributions. The programs should not be simply "nice activities" but a possibility for changing lives and communities.

The ability of community organizing to make long-term systemic change has been contested since its inception as a field. Many of the problems, which intergenerational community organizing with African Americans seeks to address, are imposed on the community from external sources. Therefore, the limited amount of change that does occur may not affect the larger systems (economic, political, educational, power, etc.) that affect communities.

In spite of these critiques, community organizing remains a popular model for improving the lives of disadvantaged residents and communities. The social problems that intergenerational community organizing with African Americans seeks to address exist in abundance within urban communities. Many of the more serious issues are untouched because of a lack of power among community residents. Intergenerational community organizing with African Americans can raise hopes and affect small incremental changes in the issues that these communities face. Systemic change often remains an elusive goal.

Further, intergenerational programming itself is not the panacea for all problems. Although these relationships are important, they must have realistic expectations of the outcomes and the work that is required. Simply placing youths and older adults in the same room will not manifest the desired outcomes (Scannell & Roberts, 1994). There has to be an opportunity for discussion, interaction, engagement, and understanding. Activities that promote more than surface contact are required to foster a safe space for the benefits of intergenerational programs to manifest. Intergenerational community organizing with African Americans is one model for a safe space.

REFERENCES

Alinsky, S. D. (1946). *Reveille for radicals* (1969 edition). New York: Random House.

Alridge, D. P. (2005). From civil rights to hip hop: Toward a nexus of ideas. *The Journal of African American History, 90*(3), 226-252.

Bankhead, T., & Erlich, J. L. (2005). Diverse populations and community practice. In M. Weil (Ed.), *The handbook of community practice* (pp. 59-83). Thousand Oaks, CA: Sage Publications.

Biklen, D. P. (1983). *Community organizing theory and practice.* Englewood Cliffs, NJ: Prentice Hall.

Carlton-LaNey, I. (Ed.) (2001). *African American leadership: An empowerment tradition in social welfare history.* Washington, DC: NASW Press.

Chaskin, R. J., Joseph, M. L., & Chipenda-Dansokho, S. (1998). Implementing comprehensive community development: Possibilities and limitations. In P. L. Ewalt, E. M. Freeman, & D. L. Poole (Eds.), *Community building: Renewal, well-being, and shared responsibility* (pp. 17-28). Washington, DC: NASW Press.

Chekki, D. A. (1979). *Community development:Theory and method of planned change.* New Delhi: Vikas.

Christenson, J. A., Fendley, K., & Robinson, J. Jr. (1989). Community development. In J. A. Christenson & J. W. Robinson Jr. (Eds.), *Community development in perspective.* Iowa: Iowa State University Press.

Cook, S. W. (2001). Mary Church Terrell and her mission: Giving decades of quiet service. In I. Carlton-LaNey (Ed.), *African American leadership: An empowerment tradition in social welfare history* (p. 153). Washington, DC: NASW Press.

Day, P. J. (2003). *A new history of social welfare* (4th ed.). Boston, MA: Allyn & Bacon.

Delgado, G. (1994). *Beyond the politics of place: New directions in community organizing in the 1990's.* Oakland, CA: Applied Research Center.

Domina, T. (2006) Brain drain and brain gain: Rising educational segregation in the United States, 1940-2000. *City & Community, 5*(4), 387-407.

Eichler, M. (1995). Consensus organizing: Sharing power to gain power. *National Civic Review, 84*(3), 256-271.

Ewalt, P. L., Freeman, E. M., & Poole, D. L. (1998). *Community building: Renewal, well-being, and shared responsibility.* Washington, DC: NASW Press.

Ganz, M. (2002). What is organizing? *Social Policy, 33*(1), 16-17.

Gilens, M. (1999). *Why Americans hate welfare.* Chicago: University of Chicago Press.

Ginwright, S. A. (2005). On urban ground: Understanding African American intergenerational partnerships in urban communities. *Journal of Community Psychology, 33*(1), 101-110.

Gittell, R., & Vidal, A. (1998). *Community organizing: Building social capital as a development strategy.* Thousand Oaks, CA: Sage Publications.

Guinier, L. (1994). *The tyranny of the majority.* New York: Basic Books.

Gutierrez, L., Alvarez, A. R., Nemon, H., & Lewis, E. A. (1996). Multicultural community organizing: A strategy for change. *Social Work, 41*(5), 501-508.

Henkin, N., & Kingson, E. (1998). Advancing an intergenerational agenda for the twenty-first century: An opportunity for compassion, respect for differences, and strong social bonds. *Generations, 22*(4), 99-106.

HoSang, D. (2003). Youth and community organizing today. *Social Policy, 34*(2/3), 66-70.

Hunt, L. (2001). Beyond cultural competence. *Religiously informed cultural competence, November/December*(24). Retrieved December 11, 2006 from http://www.parkridgecenter.org/Page1882.html.

Kahn, S. (1992). *Organizing: A guide for grassroots leaders.* New York: McGraw Hill.

Kaplan, M. (1997). The benefits of intergenerational community service projects: Implications for promoting intergenerational unity, community activism, and cultural continuity. *Journal of Gerontological Social Work, 28*(3), 211-228.

Kaplan, M., & Liu, S. (2004). *Generations united for environmental awareness and action.* Washington, DC: Generations United.

Karenga, M. (2006). *The official Kwanzaa website.* Retrieved December 11, 2006 from http://www.officialkwanzaawebsite.org/index.shtml

Katz, M. (1989). *The undeserving poor: From the war on poverty to the war on welfare.* New York: Pantheon Books.

Kirst-Ashman, K., & Hull, G. Jr. (2006). *Understanding generalist practice* (4th ed.). Pacific Grove, CA: Brooks/Cole.

Miles, T. P. (1999). Living with chronic disease and the policies that bind. In T. P. Miles (Ed.), *Full-color aging: Facts, goals, and recommendations for America's diverse elders* (pp. 53-63). Washington, DC: Gerontological Society of America.

Mondros, J. B., & Wilson, S. M. (1994). *Organizing for power and empowerment.* New York: Columbia University Press.

Northouse, P. (2003). *Leadership theory and practice* (3rd ed.). Thousand Oaks, CA: Sage Publications.

Peterman, W. (2000). *Neighborhood planning and community-based development: The potential and limits of grassroots action.* London: Sage Publications.

Pleck, E. H. (2001). Kwanzaa: An invented Black Nationalist tradition, 1966-1990. *Journal of American Ethnic History, 20,* 3-28.

Scannell, T., & Roberts, A. (1994). *Young and old serving together: Meeting community needs through intergenerational partnerships.* Washington, DC: Generations United.

Schiele, J. H. (2000). *Human services and the Afrocentric paradigm.* Binghamton, NY: The Haworth Press.

Schriver, J. M. (2004). *Human behavior and the social environment* (4th ed.). Boston: Allyn & Bacon.

Shragge, E., & Fisher, R. (2001). Community organizing: A call to action. *Canadian Dimension, 35*(2), 40.

Stoecker, R. (2003). Understanding the community development-organizing dialectic. *Journal of Urban Affairs, 25*(4), 493-512.

Stovall, D. (2006). We can relate: Hip-hop culture, critical pedagogy, and the secondary classroom. *Urban Review, 41*(6), 585-602.

Trattner, W. I. (1999). *From poor law to welfare state: A history of social welfare in America* (6th ed.). New York: Free Press.

Visser, M. J. (2004). Implementing peer support in schools: Using a theoretical framework in action research. *Journal of Community & Applied Social Psychology, 14*(6), 436-454.

Warren, M. (2001). *Dry bones rattling.* Princeton: Princeton University Press.

Family Survival:
Passing the Intergenerational Torch

Andrea Stewart

A silver haired, soft-spoken great-grandmother reached
    out for her daughter's hand to connect in love
To comfort her woes, to ease her pains, and to remind
    her of guardian angels sent from above
Of protection and guidance from day to day
    assured through a spiritual belief unexplainable
    to the average soul
Four generations united within one household
    sharing responsibilities, historical events,
    and stories yet untold
Of mutual respect, strength, individuality, collective
    bargaining and value-laden decision making
A tightly knit family, interconnected and resilient.

A beauty that is breathtaking captures inward
    and outward portrayals of family
Exhibited through energetic, charismatic,
    and intuitive children and grandchildren ranging
    in ages and physiques
Eager to voice their thoughts and concerns
    as they unconsciously embrace their parents'
    techniques and legacy
Of endurance, cooperation, co-optation, and survival
Strategies observed throughout the years emerge
    and strength-based perspectives guide family life.

Social Work Practice with African-American Families

As tears, fears, multiple problems, and crises surface,
    great-grandmother's presence merely calms everyone
    and epitomize her grace
As the family's matriarch, she is united
    with great-grandfather who is passing
    the intergenerational torch
To maintain our family's culture and survival
For our family's torch burns eternally as we embrace
    all mankind without denial
Of challenges, differences and similarities
    that truly exist.

INDEX